LIVE
IN THE
BALANCE

LINDA PROUT, M.S.

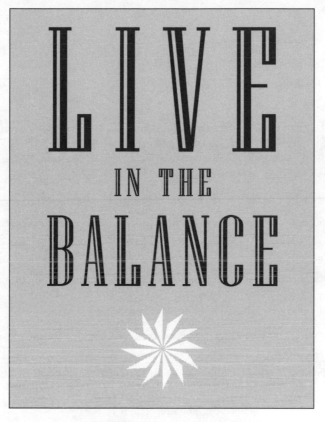

LIVE
IN THE
BALANCE

THE GROUND-BREAKING
EAST WEST
NUTRITION PROGRAM

MARLOWE & COMPANY
NEW YORK

Published by
Marlowe & Company
A Division of Avalon Publishing Group Incorporated
841 Broadway, 4th Floor
New York, NY 10003

Live in the Balance: *The Ground-Breaking East-West Nutrition Program*
Copyright © 2000 Linda Prout, M.S.

Library of Congress Cataloging-in-Publication Data
Prout Linda.
Live in the balance : the ground-breaking-East-West nutrition program / by Linda Prout.
p. cm.
Includes bibliographical references.
ISBN 1-56924-615-7
1. Nutrition. 2. Medicine, Chinese. I. Title.

RA784 .P76 2000
613.2—dc21   00-056051

9 8 7 6 5 4 3 2 1

DESIGNED BY PAULINE NEUWIRTH, NEUWIRTH & ASSOCIATES, INC.

Printed in the United States of America
Distributed by Publishers Group West

This book is dedicated to my teachers, be they clients, experts in the health profession, or healers, and to the universal energy that guides us all to heal

"Many diseases can be cured by diet alone."
—*Principles of Correct Diet*, Chinese text, 1330

CONTENTS

PREFACE

People seeking relief from chronic illness, low energy, cravings, and excess weight are drawn to my unique combination of Western nutritional science and Chinese medicine. I reach thousands of people through classes, TV, workshops, group speaking and in my private practice at the Claremont Resort and Spa in Berkeley, California. My clients often say they came to me because they are intrigued by this blend of Eastern wisdom with Western science. Most of them know a fair amount about nutrition but still can't stay with a diet or find a way of eating that provides a satisfactory level of health. By recommending specific foods and preparation techniques for specific situations and conditions, I not only help to alleviate my client's symptoms but also give them the tools they need to maintain long-term health, weight control, and energy.

I work with a surprisingly wide range of people and health dilemmas. There's the stressed-out advertising account manager who says, "I've gained fifty pounds since taking this job." She eats to calm herself at the end of the day. I'm working with a lawyer who wants off Prozac without slipping back into depression. I look forward to sessions with a grandmother who wants to know how to eat to stay mentally sharp and agile so she can enjoy her grand-children for years to come. Several clients have found relief from seasonal hay fever and allergies through a change in food choices. Another was able to come off migraine and hypertension medications and actually become free of the headaches and, for the first time in twenty-five years, lower a tenacious blood pressure problem.

Many of my clients have found relief from the bloating, cramping, diar-rhea, and constipation of bowel diseases. Women find they no longer need to suffer from PMS or menopause symptoms at midlife by simply altering their food choices.

A remarkable success involved a seventeen-year-old girl who came to me with such debilitating arthritis that she couldn't even open my office door. Her parents had to turn her over in bed at night. Her pain kept her from vir-tually any movement so she had put on 100 excess pounds. She swallowed sixteen prescribed pills each day. However, within a few months after chang-ing her food choices, her pain had eased. She was down to one pill, and she was exercising. Less than a year later, she'd lost seventy-five pounds and started a college teaching program.

My own experience taught me how the right balance of food choices and lifestyle can change one's life. A former overweight stressed-out overeater with close to 100 weight-loss diets under my belt, I was able to balance my moods, gain control over my appetite, become slender, and restore my natu-rally energetic nature by incorporating Eastern culinary wisdom with Western science.

My own mood, weight, and overeating problems started at age thirteen, about the time I started dieting. Though my weight was normal, I was con-vinced I was fat and embarked on a number of restrictive weight-loss pro-grams, including the Air Force Diet, Dr. Stillman's diet (a high-protein regi-men), a vegetarian diet, an all-fruit plan, juice fasts, a bananas-only diet, Dr. Atkins' diet, a cabbage-soup diet, and Weight Watchers. Despite protests from my mother and the luscious smells of lasagna and other goodies com-ing from the kitchen each evening, I persisted as best I could with the diet of the week. With each one, I did lose weight, but I would feel anxious and eventually go off the diet by bingeing on cookies, bread, pizza, and pasta.

The weight always seemed to come back much more quickly than it came off, leaving me a few pounds heavier each time.

By age fifteen, I was several clothing sizes larger than when I started my first diet, yet still hopeful I'd find the right regimen. It was about that time I began a vegetarian diet, focusing on lots of salads, pasta, and beans. The cravings seemed to escalate. My moods and energy levels fluctuated as radically as the diets themselves. On some days, I felt too depressed to leave my bedroom. I often shunned friends and high-school activities. Sometimes I was too tired to go to school or even have dinner out with my family, while at other times I became angry at the slightest provocation. I later realized that this erratic and unhappy behavior had much to do with my brain chemistry, which was impacted by what I was eating. I was following diets that ultimately led to insatiable urges to devour plates of pasta with garlic bread, cookies, and carrot cake, foods that left me tired and depressed.

I thought that if I could just learn more about nutrition, my problems would be solved. I was determined to discover a diet that would help me to stay slim, energized, and happy. I enrolled in one of the country's best four-year nutrition programs at the University of California at Davis. You can imagine my reaction when I saw that several of my nutrition professors were overweight, including a renowned obesity expert. In fact, many of my classmates suffered from eating disorders, either bingeing and purging or stuffing themselves between diets. One young woman was running six to seven miles a day just to "burn off all the extra food I eat." During final exams and high-stress semesters, I binged and my weight climbed; during summers, when things were more relaxed, I binged less frequently and the weight went down a bit. Eventually, I graduated—thirty pounds over my ideal weight. My belly was bloated and distended from eating so many salads, and I was still besieged by intense chocolate and sugar cravings, the very foods I knew weren't healthy. I was tired, depressed, and disillusioned.

Out of desperation I became more determined than ever to find the answers. I took on what has become a lifelong mission to find the ideal way of eating for fitness, vitality, and perfect health. As traditional Western studies offered little help for my food and mood issues, I began searching alternatives to mainstream western medicine and nutrition. I found nutrition oriented MDs who taught me how to use food and nutritional supplements to alleviate digestive problems, skin ailments, heart disease, mood disorders, and a host of other health problems. I observed how nutrition could restore balance to the body rather simply affecting the symptoms as do drugs. The adjustments I made to my own food choices began to revive my energy, yet I still wasn't feeling as good as I knew was possible.

Hungering for more information, I sought out Oriental Medical Doctors (OMDs) who taught me about Chinese medicine and nutrition. Through them I learned my cravings and fatigue had to do with an imbalance in my digestion, exacerbated by my copious intake of salads and lack of meat, fish, or poultry. Switching to more cooked vegetables and adding fish and chicken back to my diet returned to me a sense of vitality I hadn't experienced for years; one that finally quenched my insatiable need for sweets. I went on to complete a formal Traditional Chinese Medicine course series.

After using an Eastern approach to find balance for myself, I began to look at Western science in a new way. The idea of balanced brain chemistry seemed to fit with the Chinese yin/yang model of balance. With renewed energy and enthusiasm, I returned to school to get my master's degree in nutrition from the University of Connecticut at Bridgeport. My graduate research focused on the connections between food and brain chemistry and mood. I learned how brain chemistry drives our moods and cravings and how selecting the right foods at the right times can restore us to balance. It was something ancient cultures have observed for thousands of years. Upon completion of my degree, I traveled to China to observe Eastern healing firsthand. The energetic, tempered nature of the Chinese seemed to reflect their balanced food choices. Western studies of the Chinese show their heart disease, cancer, and obesity rates are a mere fraction of ours.

Once I realized the power of balancing food choices for myself, I began helping others find the best way of eating for their unique situations. Close to twenty years of feedback from clients has been an important teacher. My clients remark at their new sense of calm, the ease with which they lost weight, and their ability to get off medications, such as cholesterol-lowering drugs and antidepressants—all through nutrition.

This path of discovery has been long, fascinating, and sometimes bewildering, but it brought me the answers for which I'd long been searching. For the first time, I understand the true meaning of balance and how our poor food choices can pull us from our center and our ideal state of health and well being.

PREFACE

This book condenses many years of learning. By reading it, you will come to understand how the wrong food choices for your needs can knock you off balance and create health problems, while the right food choices can relieve health problems, boost your energy, lift your spirits, keep you fit, and bring you to a wonderfully delicious and vital place where you feel the drive and inspiration to reach your goals and live your dreams.

LIVE
IN THE
BALANCE

INTRODUCTION:
AN EAST–WEST WAY TO BALANCE

When you consider the medical advances of the last century and the state of American health today, you've got to wonder, "Where have we gone wrong?" We've spent billions of dollars researching ways to detect and treat illnesses. We've developed drugs that can arrest cancer growth and destroy once-fatal infectious organisms. We can perform microscopic surgery through barely visible incisions, restoring vision with a focused beam of light. We have more diet books, gyms, fat-free foods, and metabolism-boosting, appetite-suppressing agents than any other country in the world. Yet, look at us.

Almost half of all working American adults are in poor health, many with serious chronic conditions such as arthritis, heart and artery disease, high blood pressure, and diabetes.[1] Americans die of heart disease and certain cancers at five to thirty times the rate of people in many parts of the world.[2] Nine million Americans are taking cholesterol-lowering drugs, yet two in five Americans will die of heart disease, the nation's leading cause of death. The incidence of diabetes, the fourth-leading cause of death in the United States, is increasing: In 1900, less than 1 percent of the population had the disease, while an estimated 8 percent of us have it today.[3] We have one of the world's highest rates of obesity, and the problem is only getting worse: The percentage of obese American adults has climbed from 24 percent in the 1960s to 34 percent today. Our fatness contributes to our high blood pressure, arthritis, diabetes, and heart disease. Psychologically, we're also unwell. Approximately seventeen million Americans are clinically depressed, and more than fourteen million suffer from anxiety, with twenty-eight million taking antidepressant or anti-anxiety medication. What makes the statistics even more dismal is that we've been working so hard to overcome these health problems, to no avail.

Americans are becoming increasingly aware of the power of diet in preventing and treating disease. But we're confused. Nutrition discoveries and recommendations often seem to be contradictory. Are eggs good for us or do they clog our arteries? Is sugar a safe, fat-free carbohydrate or does it lead to disease? One week we hear about the virtues of carbohydrates and are encouraged to feast on pasta, potatoes, and bread; the next we're told to throw out the bread and bagels and replace them with meat, chicken, and other protein-rich foods to keep us in "the Zone."

We have a blind spot in our approach to diet, medicine, and health. We're missing something. The practice of nutrition in America is controversial and conflicting because we focus on one-size-fits-all remedies like loads of garlic for everyone wanting to avoid cancer or heart disease, echinecea for everyone with a cold, and low-fat diets for everyone who wants to lose weight. The truth is there are as many remedies and diets as there are people, and what works for one person won't necessarily work for the next. Just because fifty out of seventy-five people in a test study found relief or lost weight with a new drug or food program doesn't necessarily mean you will too.

THE SEARCH FOR MAGIC BULLETS

It's no secret that some foods, such as refined sugars and saturated fats, can lead to health problems. We can logically suppose that other foods improve overall health, and Western researchers have been vigorously exploring the subtle and unique healing properties of certain foods. These scientists have identified a number of vitamins, minerals, fibers, and other plant chemicals that prevent and possibly treat diseases.

Broccoli, cauliflower, and brussels sprouts, for instance, contain substances that help remove carcinogens from cells. Rice bran contains tocotrienol, a substance similar to vitamin E that may reduce cholesterol levels. Dark green leafy vegetables such as spinach, kale, and mustard-family greens are rich in folic acid, a nutrient known to reduce the risk of several diseases. In looking at 88,756 women from Harvard's Nurses' Health Study, researchers found those subjects who consumed a least 400 micrograms of folic acid daily (equivalent to about two cups of cooked spinach) over fourteen years lowered their colon cancer risk by about 75 percent. If taken in sufficient quantities by women before and during pregnancy, folic acid also reduces the risk of spina bifida, a crippling birth defect, from afflicting a fetus.

Foods such as fish, poultry, beef, and green vegetables provide amino acids, magnesium, folic acid, and other B vitamins that help our brains make enough neurotransmitters, such as serotonin, to keep our moods elevated. At a time when sales of the antidepressant drug Prozac—which functions by ensuring that serotonin levels remain relatively high—exceed $2 billion per year, eating right makes even more sense, financially and otherwise.

But while identifying individual health-promoting nutrients represents a big step toward achieving wellness, these findings illuminate only fragments of a huge health puzzle. The Western approach to nutritional research is to seek out magic bullets for specific targets. We know that the beta-carotene found in carrots and other vegetables may reduce cancer risk and that soy foods are associated with fewer cases of breast and prostate cancers among large population groups. But these findings may not be relevant to individuals like you and me, with our highly idiosyncratic systems. These studies are designed to determine how many people improve or worsen with a given food or nutrient, not to reveal the specific circumstances under which that food may be helpful nor to show you the best remedy for your unique constitution.

Take milk. As we all know, milk contains calcium, a mineral essential for building strong bones. Yet give a glass of milk to an individual who is unable to handle milk proteins or sugars (lactose), and he or she will develop debilitating stomach cramps, gas, bloating, and diarrhea. The calcium in milk—however beneficial it may be to bones—won't reach those bones if the milk itself cannot be properly digested. And think about this: Most of the world's population stops drinking milk after infancy, and yet many of those cultures maintain healthier, stronger bones than do milk-drinking cultures.

When studying nutritional treatments, scientists are looking for statistical significance within a select research population. They try to determine what percentage of a group of volunteers are positively affected by a diet or a specific nutrient. If anything less than a *significant majority* of research participants are helped by a nutrient or diet, the tested food or program is considered an "unproven remedy," even if some of the participants experienced real improvements in their health. Unfortunately, these kinds of studies ignore meaningful associations between different types of constitutions, ailments, and food remedies.

WHY EXTREME DIETS FAIL

The fallout from this fragmented way of researching nutrition is an unbalanced way of eating. In the quest to feel and look better, Americans have tried to integrate scientific findings into all sorts of extreme diets. Swinging like a pendulum, we've gone from high-fat, protein-rich diets to low-fat, high-carbohydrate diets and back again over the past few decades. We seem inexorably drawn to the next diet, the best food, the quick fix for our ailing hearts and expanding waistlines.

Such extreme diets are doomed to fail because they create imbalance. High-protein regimens lead to cravings, and more than 90 percent of the time the weight is ultimately regained, while high-carbohydrate systems leave us fatigued and fatter. Our health doesn't improve and we don't lose weight, in part because it's impossible to adhere to these programs. The longer we stay on them, the more we feel out of control. And, in the end, without balance in nutrition we have a greater susceptibility to illness, depression, and anxiety. Before we can understand how to balance our diets for optimum health and weight, let us explore further how and why extreme diets fail, even though they are often based on or seem to coincide with scientific findings.

High-Carbohydrate Diets

At present, the Government-espoused view on nutrition is that a high-carbohydrate, low-fat, and, consequently, low-protein diet is best. For everyone.

Many health experts consider carbohydrates such as pasta, cereals, breads, and potatoes—even cookies, sorbet, and candy, as long as they are low fat or fat free—to be wholesome alternatives to meats and other animal products. According to this perspective, carbohydrates should form the foundation of a healthful diet. And indeed, this thinking is supported by the government-sponsored food pyramid, which recommends that we eat six to eleven servings of carbohydrate-rich foods daily.

Fat in this system is thought to be "bad." And sure enough, countless studies show that eating too much fat can clog your arteries, increase cancer risks, and make you obese. Fat's accomplice, protein, is also linked with disease. High-protein diets, according to some researchers, may lead to heart disease, certain cancers, and kidney disease. Since it's difficult to separate fat from protein in the foods we eat and many cuts of meat, poultry, eggs, cheese, and some fish are high in both, advocates for high-carbohydrate diets believe the excess meat, cheese, and eggs we've been eating during the past century have caused the enormous rise in heart disease and reshaped us into "apples." These people, some of whom have written best-selling books on the subject, promote virtually fat-free, low-protein, meatless eating as the way to achieve heart health, long lives, and ideal weight.

If you've been following the traditional American meat-, cheese-, and butter-rich diet for a while, or if a protein-rich, high-fat diet disagrees with you, fat-free or low-fat eating feels wonderful at first. It's a powerful medicine that almost immediately balances years of excessive, heavy protein and fat eating. High cholesterol levels often begin to drop, excess weight begins to fall, and flagging energy levels are revived. This taste of health leads many to believe they've found the perfect life-long plan.

However, after it takes you to the point of balance, fat-free, low-protein eating often begins to weaken the body. Scientific studies show we need some fats—specifically, essential fats—and after a period of avoiding all fats we begin to crave fatty foods to fulfill these needs. A fat deficiency can lead to a number of common health problems, including skin problems, arthritis, diabetes, obesity, high blood pressure, heart disease, and depression. Some of us need more fat or protein than others do to stay healthy, but even if you fare best with low fat foods, deficiencies of fat-soluble vitamins such as A, D, and E may eventually develop on such a diet. Your immunity may drop, allowing for greater risk of colds and infections. Your skin may become dry and flaky, and your hair may begin to look dull. Arthritic inflammation may set into your joints. In women, premenstrual symptoms may worsen. With a fat deficiency, you experience cravings for cookies, sweet rolls, and excess bread. Your energy level plummets. Eventually even body weight begins to climb back up. (Of course, such symptoms flare up more quickly and severely in those who have a greater requirement for essential fats than others do.) Ironically, the very low-fat diets that initially help us fight excess weight and a host of diseases ultimately contribute to some of the same health problems.

High-Protein Diets

If extreme high-carbohydrate diets are not the answer to better health and optimum weight, what about high-protein programs? Every bit as popular as the high-carb regimens, if not as widely accepted by conventional health authorities, are the high-protein ones. Advocates of this nutrition stance claim that fat- and protein-rich diets are going to save us from heart disease, diabetes, obesity, and premature death. The doctors who authored many of the popular protein-touting diet books on the market today say too many plates of spaghetti, slices of bread, bowls of corn flakes, and other carbs are leading us down the path to disease, fatigue, and love handles.

High-protein supporters recommend a diet rich in meat, eggs, cheese, butter, and oils but limited in sugar, fruit, grains, bread, and pasta. Protein-rich foods such as meat, fish, and eggs can indeed be powerful medicine, especially for certain conditions. Anemia can be alleviated by increasing the amount of meat in one's diet. Some individuals find if they don't regularly consume fish, chicken, beef, or other animal protein, they are plagued by fatigue and indigestion. Athletes and those who engage in regular vigorous activity generally find animal protein gives them more vigor and stamina. Weight watchers enjoy greater satiety and often faster weight loss with the appropriate type and amount of protein foods in their diet than they do on high-carbohydrate, meatless fare. Much of the weight loss associated with very high-protein diets unfortunately occurs in large part from loss of water, not fat, since high-protein diets are dehydrating—potentially dangerously so. Moreover, eating a lot of high-protein foods places an extra load on the kidneys, which must work harder to eliminate the excess nitrogen found in meats.

In touting the benefits of high-meat diets, protein proponents cite something called "the glycemic index," a measure of how high a particular food sends up sugar levels in the bloodstream, which in turn trigger the release of the hormone insulin from the pancreas. Insulin maintains an appropriate range of sugars in the blood by helping to direct the transportation of sugars from the bloodstream into liver and muscle cells, which either use the sugars to produce energy or store them for future use. Unlike steak, eggs, and beans, many carbohydrates—especially white bread, many breakfast cereals, jelly beans, and cookies—generally have high glycemic index values. They trigger a rise in blood sugar and, the reasoning goes, in the corresponding insulin levels, because more insulin is needed to get the high amount of sugars either used or stored in the body's cells, thus keeping sugar levels down in the bloodstream. High levels of insulin tend to promote fat storage in adipose cells on your hips, thighs, and elsewhere, increasing the risk of diabetes and heart disease.

Some research, however, conflicts with the idea that simple carbohydrate foods have a higher glycemic index than protein foods. According to Jeffrey Bland, PhD, founder and director of HealthComm International Clinical Research Center, some fatty foods, including fried foods, may have a higher glycemic index than some carbohydrate foods. In addition, some people experience a higher glycemic index and greater insulin release with certain foods than others do. For example, steak, a high-protein food, generally has a low glycemic index and thus should be helpful for blood-sugar control and energy-level boosts. Yet in some people, steak triggers the opposite reaction: Blood sugar drops, insulin levels rise, fatigue sets in, and the pounds can build up again. One person's meat is another person's poison.

While certain fat-rich foods, including fatty fish, some seeds, and nuts, can help burn fat and protect against heart disease, other types of fats found in a high-protein diet are detrimental to our health. The saturated fats in whole-milk products, beef, pork, and other animal foods may contribute to elevated cholesterol levels, the build-up of sticky plaque occluding the arteries, and thicker blood which has a greater tendency to clot. All these factors lead to greater risk of heart attack. Cutting back on saturated fat-rich meats, cheese, and butter may lower elevated blood-cholesterol levels by 10 to 20 percent. By reducing meats and fat-containing dairy products, cholesterol *intake* is also reduced, potentially reducing blood-cholesterol levels and thus the risk of heart disease even more in some people. (For most people, cholesterol intake has no effect on blood cholesterol levels.) Saturated fats and even high levels of protein itself are also associated with the increased cancer rates. Advanced prostate tumors in men are six times more likely in the United States than in Japan, where fat intake is roughly half ours.

High-protein diets also increase calcium excretion, thereby contributing to bone loss and the resulting condition of osteoporosis. Within two to four hours after high-protein foods such as meat enter your system, your blood becomes more acidic; an acidic environment prevents calcium from being optimally retained and absorbed into bones, and more of it than usual is released in the urine. A low- or moderate-protein, vegetable-rich diet, on the other hand, helps the body absorb calcium, which aids in building or maintaining bone strength.

The bottom line is that high-protein diets are not viable for most people in the long run. Like high-carbohydrate diets, they are unbalanced, especially in those people who fare better with more plant foods.

ANCIENT SOLUTIONS FOR MODERN PROBLEMS

Despite our sophisticated medical technology and extensive research on specific nutrients, we are still overweight and prone to serious diseases. The worn-out high-carbohydrate and high-protein diets and the single-nutrient, magic-bullet strategies clearly are not working for us. We need a fresh perspective on food and health, one that recognizes our different nutritional needs and takes into account the subtle interplay of environmental, emotional, and physiological factors in determining those needs. We can find such a perspective in China, a country that is relatively free of the diseases killing us—a country whose people stay slim though they eat more than we do.

By comparing principles of Chinese culinary practices with emerging Western studies, we are beginning to see areas of common ground, despite the cultural differences. The Chinese approach shows us how to apply the unique healing properties of everyday foods to balance common health problems. Western science supports these observations with recent discoveries of healing nutrients and phytochemicals.

Since 1983, T. Collin Campbell, PhD, a nutritional biochemist at Cornell University, and Dr. Chen Junshi, of the Chinese Institute of Nutrition and Food Hygiene in Beijing, have been studying the eating habits and health of 6,500 people in sixty-four counties across China. Called the China–Cornell–Oxford Diet and Health Project, Campbell and Junshi's study has given us an inside look at the dietary habits of a population that is relatively free of the diseases plaguing Western societies.

Centuries of observation have guided the Chinese to a vegetable-based diet, one Americans have only relatively recently discovered reduces risk of disease and prolongs life. The Chinese eat 30 percent more calories than we do and skip the gym workout, yet they are 25 percent thinner than we are. On top of that, say the Cornell researchers, the Chinese have seventeen times fewer cases of heart disease, one-fifth the rate of breast cancer, and less than half the instances of colon cancer we do. Their cholesterol levels are about half ours. These kinds of findings have researchers looking at the millennia-old principles of Traditional Chinese Medicine (TCM) for answers to our health issues.

Numerous Western studies verify that a Chinese–style, plant-based diet protects against the leading causes of death in this country (heart disease, cancer, and stroke) and helps normalize weight. The traditional Chinese diet also helps facilitate a greater sense of calm and fewer emotional swings than does a meat-centered or refined carbohydrate-centered diet. A relaxed, balanced emotional state is associated with improved immunity, better brain function, and enhanced memory, as well as lower risk of heart disease, cancer, ulcers, and stroke. A sense of calm also helps keep appetite normal and minimizes the cravings that can lead to overeating and obesity.

The Chinese liberal vegetable intake provides many times the magnesium as the typical American diet does. Magnesium, a nutrient found in plant foods, especially nuts, sea vegetables, leafy greens, and whole grains, controls a protein in the brain that contributes to anxiety.[4] Research indicates a magnesium-rich diet lowers blood pressure, perhaps because of its ability to instill calm.[5] Magnesium also reduces risk of stroke, which often occurs when we experience periods of extreme anxiety.

The Chinese also consume a substantial amount of broccoli-family vegetables, including cabbage, cauliflower, and kale, which provide sulfur-containing substances (*sulforaphane*) that reduce the risk of cancer. Their daily intake of bok choy, kale, spinach, chinese broccoli (*gai lan*), pea sprouts, and other dark leafy greens deliver nutrients—such as folic acid—necessary for elevating mood and boosting energy as well as protecting the body from heart disease, cancer, and stroke. Folic acid prevents the build-up of a chemical called *homocysteine* in the blood. Recent studies have linked high homocysteine levels with increased risk of heart disease. Women also need sufficient levels of folic acid in order to prevent spinal defects in their offspring. US diets don't contain the levels of folic acid needed to protect against heart disease and spinal defects.[6]

The Chinese are also great drinkers of green tea: Throughout the cities and villages of China, people can be seen carrying jars of green tea leaves, replenishing them with hot water wherever they go. Green tea may be one of the cheapest, most practical ways to prevent cancer in the general population, according to researchers in this country.[7] A generous intake of green tea protects against cancers of the stomach, lung, and skin as well as reduces heart disease and obesity. Green tea contains a substance called *epigallocatechin gallate* (EGCG), a constituent of tannin that limits the growth of cancer cells. It also appears to control blood cholesterol levels and to prevent blood from becoming sticky and forming clots.

And, of course, the Chinese eat a lot of soy-based foods. According to Western research, foods such as tofu, tempeh, and miso soup play a role in reducing breast and prostate cancers and heart disease. Studies show soy foods also help balance hormone levels and are thus major allies in keeping menopause symptoms to a minimum. Studies of Japanese women—who, like the Chinese, have a high intake of soy products—report a tenfold decrease in reported hot flashes. The Japanese also have one quarter the incidence of heart disease of Americans.[8] A number of studies have shown regular intake of soy products reduces cholesterol levels, particularly the most harmful LDL type, while increasing the beneficial HDL levels.[9]

The Chinese system combines these types of foods, plus herbs, into a complete eating strategy for each individual's unique needs. This strategy is more complex than the Western approach of singling out specific nutrients for specific diseases. Despite all the great health-promoting advantages of tofu, for instance, this soy food is considered very "cooling" to the system, and eating it regularly may further imbalance someone who tends to feel cold, leading to anemia, indigestion, abdominal bloating, and loose stools. To correct or prevent such problems, the Chinese carefully combine foods with those qualities that will restore or maintain balance for the individual in question. Additionally, illnesses and symptoms are treated with remedies that balance the underlying condition. Someone with high blood pressure, a hot temper, a flushed face, and arthritis, for example, is treated for the entire set of problems and tendencies, not just the conditions of arthritis and high blood pressure. His or her food remedy assuages the tendency toward anger, cools the redness of skin, and reduces the inflammation in the joints.

In China, food and healing are inseparable, and cooking is a highly sophisticated art form that balances flavors and other properties of foods to harmonize the body. This book draws upon the wisdom of this extraordinary healing tradition and combines that wisdom with state-of-the-art western science. In reading the following chapters, you will learn the basic principles of Chinese nutrition, determine your particular patterns of imbalances and discover your unique nutritional needs, and learn about the foods and cooking strategies best suited to you. By eating the foods appropriate for your constitution and set of symptoms, you will assimilate food better, and your metabolism, energy, and health will improve.

As you learn to balance yourself, keep in mind that just as individuals vary tremendously, so do your own nutritional needs, depending on the season, your age, your emotional state, your physical environment, and other factors. The foods that work for you at one time may not be right for you at another time. Unlike many other health and diet books, this book does not offer a quick fix, nor does it prescribe a single regimen for all people. Rather, it will guide you to the best nutritional choices for who and where you are right now. While no two people have exactly the same constitutions, and your own needs shift over time, one thing is certain: By following the powerful, field-tested middle path of Chinese nutrition, you will find the way to better health, improved mood and energy levels, greater satisfaction with meals, and increased ease in shedding excess pounds. And no matter what particular foods you may require, you will find that balance is the secret ingredient that makes your diet work for you.

1. Murray, Michael, and Joseph Pizzorno, *Encyclopedia of Natural Medicine*. New York: Prima, (1998):11.
2. *Newsweek*, November 30, 1998.
3. Steward, H. Leighton, Bethea, Morrison C., Andrews, Sam W. and Balart, Luis A. *Sugar Busters*, New York: Ballantine Books, (1998): p79-80.
4. Marx, J. "Anxiety Petide Found in Brain," *Science*, (1985): 227:934.
5. Mizushimi, S., et al., "Dietary Magnesium Intake and Blood Pressure," *Hypertension* xii (1998): 447-53.
6. Durand, P., et al., "Folate Deficiencies and Dardiovasular Pathologies," *Clinical Chemical Laboratory Medicine*, 36(7) (1998): 419-429
7. Fujiki, H. et al., "Cancer Inhabition by Green Tea," *Mutation Research* (1998) 402: 307–10.
8. Johnson, K. "HRT Adjuncts Include Soy, Flaxseed, Fish Oil," *Family Practice News*, November 1, 1998: 38.
9. Potter, S. M., "Soy Protein and Cardiovascular Disease: The Impact of Bioactive Components in Soy," *Nutrition Reviews* 56(8) (August 1998): 231–35.

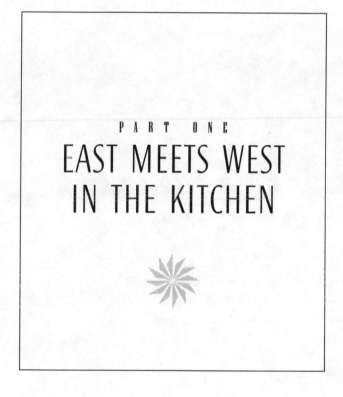

PART ONE
EAST MEETS WEST IN THE KITCHEN

I

A FRESH PERSPECTIVE:
BALANCING WHO YOU ARE
WITH WHAT YOU EAT

Because nutritional science and cuisine are still relatively young, we're just beginning to understand the properties of different foods and how they erode or contribute to overall health. In contrast, the Chinese have for thousands of years observed the ways in which specific foods, herbs, and cooking methods affect different types of people and ailments, and they have used their observations successfully to prevent and cure many health problems. China's moderate-protein, plant-based diet has protected its population from diabetes, arthritis, heart disease, cancer, and stroke—the last three being the leading causes of death in America. Yet until recently, for reasons partly cultural and partly scientific, Western nutritionists have been reluctant to take valuable cues from their Chinese counterparts. But Americans are finally beginning to pay attention to China's vast and sophisticated culinary expertise. By opening our minds to this ancient healing tradition, we are learning how to prevent and treat the diseases and weight problems that have been plaguing us, despite all our best efforts.

BALANCE: THE TAO OF HEALTH

In China, the key to health and well-being on every level is balance. Traditional Chinese Medicine (TCM) is based on ancient Taoist teachings, which speak of balance and harmony. Balance is the point of greatest strength: Riding a bicycle is impossible without a sense of balance; the martial artist attains the power to overcome an opponent by moving through the *dan tian*, the body's exact center and place of balance. Though it is a subtle concept that may not at first impress us with its muscularity—especially those of us who are used to aggressive tactics with immediate results—balance offers great power: Power for healing disease, power for controlling weight, and power over emotional ebbs and flows.

When balanced, we are filled with vitality, enthusiasm, and a sense of purpose. We have renewed patience for challenges in our work and relationships. With balance, our energy is up, but we are not anxious. Rather, we're relaxed and invigorated, clearheaded, and focused. Work tasks take less time and we make fewer mistakes. When we are in balance, we experience deep satisfaction. We lose our cravings for sweets or salty snacks, and our appetites are only for the kinds and amounts of foods that will keep us feeling in balance.

Though anyone anywhere can achieve balance, regardless of whether they are familiar with Chinese philosophy, having a basic understanding of the concepts of *yin/yang* and *Qi* will make the idea and purpose of balance that much clearer to you.

Yin and Yang

According to TCM, the forces of yin and yang combine to form everything in existence. We experience these forces as opposing qualities—cold and hot, dark and light, wet and dry, feminine and masculine—yet they are complements as well as opposites. They are descriptive terms that apply to animals, plants, people, climate, moods, food, emotions, medicine, and disease—anything you can think of can be described as relatively yin or yang. A healthy body, mind, and spirit are in dynamic balance with the yin and yang of the earth and universe. Understanding the ever-changing interplay of these polarities can help us achieve physical health, emotional well-being, personal satisfaction, and ideal weight.

The Chinese symbol, or character, for yin originated in observations of the shady side of a hill and that for yang, the sunny side of a hill. Yin qualities, then, tend to be those associated with a shady, cool place: Darkness, dampness, cold, silence, and stillness. Yang qualities, on the other hand, are those associated with a sunny place: Heat, brightness, dryness, and activity. Winter is yin while summer is yang. A foggy, cool morning is yin compared to a sunny, warm afternoon, which is yang. A woman is yin relative to a man, who is yang—or, more accurately, femininity is yin compared to masculinity, which is yang. Estrogen is a yin hormone compared to testosterone, which is a male, and therefore yang, hormone. Meditation and yoga are yin relative to football, which is yang. Compared to the stillness of meditation, however, active forms of yoga are yang.

Even moods can be relatively yin or yang. Introspection, quiet reflection, sadness, and apathy are yin states while extroversion, excitement, anxiety, and anger are yang. While these designations may sound obscure, they actually make sense from a Western scientific perspective: Melancholy and depression are more frequently associated with an excess of the female hormone estrogen (yin), whereas anger is more often associated with the male hormone, testosterone (yang). In Western cultures, we tend to value the yang qualities of aggressiveness, productivity, and vigorous activity over the yin tendencies of passivity and contemplation. The reverse is true in traditional Eastern cultures, where receptivity, patience, and meditation are encouraged and esteemed.

Yin and yang can be viewed as parts of a cycle: Spring turns into summer, day turns into night, activity turns into quiet and rest, the heat of fever turns into chills, the rigid control of dieting often turns into an out-of-control binge. The life cycle of plants begins with a tiny seed, dormant and still (yin), yet when planted in the dark moisture of the earth, the seed bursts into life and reaches for the warmth and light of the sun (yang). The active vibrancy of youth, a yang quality, slowly changes to the more yin quiescence of old age and, eventually, to the quiet darkness of death, the most yin state. As depicted by the yin/yang symbol—in which a tiny portion of yin exists within yang and a drop of yang resides within yin—everything holds the seed of its oppo-

site: We perceive light only in contrast to darkness; we understand the masculine in relation to the feminine; we know when we are sick by having experienced some degree of health.

Life Energy: Qi

Another critical concept in TCM is the notion of an invisible energy
called *Qi* (pronounced CHEE), translated as "vital force" or "life essence."
This force is said to permeate everything—all forms of life are manifesta-
tions of Qi. Life is Qi condensing, and death is its dispersal. The concept of
Qi circulating through the body is central to Chinese medicine, and our Qi
is an indication of our state of physical, mental, and spiritual health. Good
Qi shows up as vitality. According to Giovanni Maciocia in *Foundations of
Chinese Medicine*, "Qi is the root of a human being."[14]

Qi has its own movement, yet it also generates movement in organs of the
body. Western science can give a detailed explanation of how blood is
pumped through the heart, but it can't explain how this life-giving process is
perpetuated or why the heart can suddenly give out. What breathes life into
us? Why does an apparently healthy, normally functioning heart suddenly
stop beating? According to Chinese thought, Qi keeps the heart pumping,
the blood circulating, the nerves firing, the mind focused, the emotions balanced, and the digestive system functioning. To be healthy, our Qi must circulate unimpeded through our blood stream, nervous system, and organs.

Qi has several forms and functions in the body. Nutritive Qi, or *Ying Qi*
in Chinese, comes from our food and nourishes the body. As you will learn
in the next chapter, Qi from digestion (spleen Qi) transforms food into nutritive Qi, which circulates to all parts of the body for nourishment and energy. (Interestingly, the Chinese symbol for Qi is steam rising from a pot of
cooking rice.) Qi maintains the shape and perpetual motion of our organs
and keeps blood in its vessels. Qi keeps us warm and prevents us from
sweating when we're not hot. It protects us from infection.

Qi is both material and immaterial. It is matter and energy. Other cultures
also acknowledge this life energy. In our own culture, quantum physics is
tapping into the concept of Qi through the discovery that matter and energy
are interchangeable and alternate descriptions of one another. Einstein
termed this force as "subtle energy," something unable to be measured. This

matter/energy phenomenon forms the basis of certain types of healing. Deepak Chopra describes this force in his book *Quantum Healing*.[15] Leonard Laskow, MD, author of *Healing With Love* bases his noninvasive healing work on subtle energy.[16] According to Chinese medicine, we are a manifestation of our Qi. When Qi is vital and strong and unobstructed, we look vibrant, our minds are clear, and we are free of illness.

As it moves through the body, Qi can take on different forms of varying densities. When the circulation of this energy is blocked, Qi can become "stuck," manifesting as lumps or tumors. If "dampness"—a yin condition, often brought on by eating too many damp foods, such as ice cream, fried or greasy foods, and raw fruits—settles into the digestive system, Qi can be blocked, and abdominal disease or symptoms arise. Remedying such health problems requires reducing the eating and behavior patterns that lead to Qi stagnation. For example, liver Qi stagnation, which can lead to anger, mood swings, red swollen eyes, headaches, muscle stiffness, and a host of other unhealthful conditions, can occur when someone overeats, consumes too much meat or too many fried foods, drinks too much alcohol, or is plagued by long periods of stress or frustration in his or her life. By eating less, cutting back on meats, fried foods, and alcohol, and taking time off work, one can get the Qi moving from the liver and find balance.

Qi and its relation to health are discussed in much more depth in chapter three.

FINDING BALANCE THROUGH FOOD

In his book *Human Motivation and Emotion*, Ross Buck says the desire for balance lies at the root of our behavior.[17] We want it so much that when we feel out of balance—say, when we're tired, overworked, or deficient in a nutrient—we may overeat or reach for alcohol, tobacco, or sex in an attempt to feel good again. But there is a healthier way to find this balance.

Rather than focusing on radical diets to lose weight and cure illnesses, the Chinese approach to diet is to avoid food-related diseases and weight problems in the first place. "Chinese medicine embraces the logic that the best remedy for calamity is to avert it—the best cure for sickness is prevention," says Harriet Beinfield in *Between Heaven and Earth*.[18] According to the ancient medical classic *Nei Jing*, written in the second century BC, "Maintaining order rather than correcting disorder is the ultimate principle of wisdom. To cure disease after it has appeared is like digging a well when one already feels thirsty."

Learning to choose the appropriate foods for your current state helps keep you in balance. The wrong food choice, even if it is considered healthy by Western science, may leave you feeling unsatisfied, tired, anxious, irritable, or craving more of the wrong foods.

Achieving and maintaining physical and emotional balance requires a blend of whole foods that harmonize with the individual. Traditional Chinese meals focus on whole plant foods, including vegetables, beans, sea vegetables, rice, millet, and other grains, with smaller amounts of meat, poultry, and fish than are found in the typical American diet. Animal products and fat are concentrated foods, according to TCM, so although need for meats, poultry, dairy, oils, and other such foods varies from individual to individual, it generally takes smaller amounts of these foods than of plant foods for balance. (In addition, specific choices of animal foods may be poor choices for balance in certain individuals.)

Additionally, while Western food science focuses on isolating and counting phytochemicals, antioxidants, fat and protein grams, carbohydrates, and calories and then incorporating these measurements into diet regimens, traditional Chinese nutrition is based on a balance of less tangible qualities in foods: How *warming* or *cooling* they are, how *damp* or *drying* they are, and whether they can move energy, or Qi. Chinese cuisine is an art that balances the flavors, textures, and colors of foods, in turn imparting balance to those who partake. Meals and medicine in the Chinese tradition are one.

Finding the right Chinese food remedies requires reading the subtle signs and symptoms of the individual being treated, then making a correction through food and, to a lesser degree, lifestyle. The treatment might be a matter of choosing foods to enhance or lessen a mood state or to balance an environmental extreme. In effect, TCM attempts to balance who you are with what you eat.

Balancing Yin and Yang

TCM sees diseases, weight problems, and disturbing emotional and mental states as either deficiencies or excesses of yin or yang. By identifying the nature of the imbalance, one can then choose the appropriate food remedy to balance the dynamic signs. An excess yang condition can be balanced or treated by reducing yang foods, adding more yin foods and seasonings, and altering one's lifestyle or environment. The treatment balances the whole person, rather than merely alleviating the symptoms of one specific condition. When the person, rather than the disease, is treated, the odds of true healing are much greater.

For example, an overworked, agitated, middle-aged man suffering from high blood pressure, elevated cholesterol, a heated temper, and stress headaches (all yang conditions) will find relief with cooling, soothing, yin foods, including spinach, cucumbers, melon, and mushrooms. He will feel best by limiting his intake of heating, yang foods such as fried meats, spicy foods, and alcohol. Lifestyle changes might include extra time off for a vacation someplace relaxing, daily walks near a lake or in a shady park, and a program of stretching, meditation, or yoga. With these changes, his calm is easily restored, his anxiety and irritability are diminished, and his blood pressure is likely to return to normal.

On the other hand, a chilled, pale, anemic young woman will find new strength and energy and add blush to her cheeks with the addition of warming foods such as lamb stew or gingery beef. She will feel better by replacing raw salads and fruits with more cooked vegetables, especially mustard greens, onions, leeks, and garlic. She might benefit from a vigorous form of exercise, such as mountain biking or dancing.

Even if you're not unbalanced, becoming familiar with the yin and yang properties of foods can help you to feel better and be more effective on a daily basis. Need to feel strong and assertive for a job interview or presentation? Make sure to have chicken, beef, or other yang foods for lunch, and skip the fruit—too yin. Relief from the heat of a blistering summer afternoon can be found through cooling foods such as cucumber slices, cool mint tea, and watermelon. Garlic or ginger cooked into a lamb dish provides warmth for someone chilled from being outdoors on a cold winter day.

Though everyone has elements of both yin and yang, each of us can be broadly categorized as either yin or yang. A relatively yang type tends to be larger, stronger, and more muscular, with a propensity for physical activity and an assertive, gregarious nature. Unbalanced with an excess of yang, he may have a volatile temper and suffer from headaches or high blood pressure. A more yin type, on the other hand, is smaller, softer, and less toned, with a tendency to be gentle, soft-spoken, patient, and nurturing. Out of balance, the yin type tends to be soft, fleshy, and overweight and may suffer from depression, moodiness, and fatigue. A large, muscular woman is yang relative to a smaller, fleshy woman. Yet that same woman is yin compared to a larger, more muscular man.

The following thumbnail sketches of yin and yang body patterns will give you a head start in discovering your basic type. Even if you find that you fall somewhere between the two types, chances are you'll recognize yourself more in one than the other. The chapters in Part Two of this book go into depth about the many variations possible within the broad spectrum of yin and yang body patterns.

YIN BODY PATTERN

tendency to feel cold

soft voice

pale complexion

sweet taste in mouth

preference for warm foods and drinks

tendency toward loose stool

weak, soft muscles

inactive, slow

shy, insecure

quiet, still

tendency toward depression

YANG BODY PATTERN

tendency to feel warm

loud voice

red complexion

bitter taste in mouth, bad breath

preference for cold food and drink

tendency toward constipation

toned muscles

active, quick

assertive, extroverted

tendency toward mania

tendency toward anger

ORGANIC FOOD AND CHINESE NUTRITION

Organic foods should be chosen over conventionally grown foods whenever possible. Not only are organic foods less likely to harbor toxins, but also, as some studies suggest, they are more nutritious, with greater levels of vitamins and minerals. The toxins that enter our food supply through inorganic foods include herbicides, insecticides, fungicides, and heavy metals.

Antibiotics and steroid hormones come to our plates in poultry and beef as they are added to the feed of animals to prevent infections and increase their weight. Researchers have discovered the resulting human ingestion of these antibiotics reduces the effectiveness of antibiotic therapy. Overuse of antibiotics is also allowing for the growth of huge populations of new antibiotic-resistant bacteria to the environment.

The sex hormones added to animal feed to promote growth and for breeding purposes results in human hormonal imbalances, which may lead to a number of health problems, including early maturity in children, excess weight gain, infertility, kidney disease, hypertension, and cancer.[19]

Pesticides and other environmental toxins weren't an issue in ancient China. The Eastern system of diagnosis and use of various foods along with plant, animal, and mineral medicines have only recently begun to address the problems associated with toxins. Generally, the resulting patterns from excess toxins are dampness and heat (both discussed in chapter five). Toxins must pass through the liver and so place a heavy burden on this organ and may result in signs of a heated liver, including elevated liver enzymes, anger, irritability, and general moodiness.

The best ways to minimize your exposure to these toxins is to consume organic produce whenever possible and to choose range-fed, antibiotic-free poultry and beef and range-fed chicken eggs. In addition, avoid high-fat animal products such as whole milk and fatty cuts of meat since many toxins accumulate in animal fats. The Environmental Working Group, a nonprofit environmental research organization, reports that currently the twelve worst-contaminated produce items are strawberries, bell peppers, spinach, cherries, peaches, Mexican cantaloupes, celery, apples, apricots, green beans, Chilean grapes, and cucumbers.[20] My suggestion is to find these products in organic form if you want to eat them; otherwise, choose other produce.

---

14. Maciocia, Giovanni, *Foundations of Chinese Medicine*. London: Churchill Livingstone, 1989.
15. Chopra, Deepak, *Quantum Healing*. New York: Bantam, 1989.
16. Laskow, Leonard, *Healing With Love*. New York: HarperCollins, 1992.
17. Buck, Ross, *Human Motivation and Emotion*. New York: John Wiley & Sons, 1988.
18. Beinfield, Harriet, *Between Heaven and Earth*. New York: Ballantine Books, 1991.
19. Schell, Orville, *Modern Meat*. New York: Vintage Books, 28–40.
20. Ibid.

2

THE FIVE ELEMENT THEORY:
BALANCED MEALS
FOR PLEASURE AND HEALTH

Though our meal choices may be based in part on dietary or nutritional concerns, the fact is we usually select foods for the way they look on the plate and taste and feel in our mouths. We enjoy the dark, rich flavor of morning java on our tongues. We bite into a hamburger for the tantalizing blend of saltiness from the meat and cheese, sweetness of the tomato, sourness of the pickle, and pungency of the onion or mustard, and we savor the contrasting textures of the soft bread, the juicy, tender meat, and the crisp pickle and lettuce. A fresh-baked blueberry pie, with its deep-purple filling and golden-brown crust topped with silky, cloud-white whipped cream, pleases our eyes as well as our palates.

The attractive qualities of food, however, reach far beyond our eyes and our taste buds. They also have experiential qualities, such as coolness and calm, or warmth and stimulation; some correspond to the movement of vital energy, or Qi. Our desire for certain foods may have as much to do with the effects of their flavors on our organs as their sensory appeal to our tongues, and our taste preferences are often unknowingly for food combinations that are good for us. According to the Chinese Five Element Theory, meals with balanced flavors, colors, and textures not only look and taste best but also are the most satisfying and nutritionally sound. While Western nutritionists tout the healing abilities of individual nutrients, the Chinese consider a food's flavor to possess medicinal properties in and of itself, apart from its nutritional content. Interestingly, however, the foods that Western nutritionists often recommend for a certain condition on the basis of their nutrients are the same foods recommended by the Chinese for that condition by virtue of their flavors and other sensory properties. This chapter introduces you to the five elements and their corresponding bodily organs, flavors, colors, seasons, and moods. Once we know more about how each of these elements affect us and why we crave certain flavors and avoid others, we can begin to make more conscious, healthful, and satisfying meal choices.

UNDERSTANDING THE FIVE ELEMENTS OF NUTRITION

Together with yin/yang, the Chinese Five Element Theory forms the basis for TCM. Under the theory, all dimensions of life—organs, foods, colors, sounds, orientations, emotions, seasons—fit in one interconnected system. Each component relates to, and affects, another part of the system. Flavor, of course, plays a major role in Chinese nutrition. TCM recognizes five tastes, which in turn relate to five colors, five organ systems, five bodily tissues, five emotions, five environmental influences, five seasons, and five elements. When all of these components are balanced in an individual, he or she will experience good physiological, emotional, and mental health. The Five Element Theory is depicted in the diagram below.

Table of Five Elements

	ELEMENTS				
	Wood	**Fire**	**Earth**	**Metal**	**Water**
COMPONENTS					
Yin organ	liver	heart/mind	spleen	lungs	kidneys
Yang organ	gallbladder	small intestine	stomach	large intestine	bladder
Tissue	tendons	blood vessels	muscles/flesh	skin/hair	bones and sinews
Emotion	anger	joy	worry	grief	fear
Environmental Influence	wind	heat	dampness	dryness	cold
Season	spring	summer	late summer	autumn	winter
Color	green	red	yellow	white	black/dark
Flavor	sour	bitter	sweet	pungent	salty

The five elements are interconnected, with each one nourishing or controlling another. The five-element cycle, depicted below, illustrates these relationships. The clockwise direction shows the nourishing cycle: Wood burns to feed fire; fire leaves behind ashes, which become earth; earth contributes metals, which nourish water; and water stimulates the growth of plants, or wood, the beginning point on the nourishment cycle. In the controlling cycle: Wood is controlled, or cut, by metal; metal is melted by fire; fire is put out by water; water is contained and controlled by earth; and earth is taken up by wood. The controlling cycle keeps the system in check by controlling each element. The flavor of wood, which is sour, helps balance excessive use of the sweet flavor associated with the earth. The warm, energizing nature of the sweet flavor from the earth element balances a weak water element, or kidney function. Too much, or not enough, of any one flavor can lead to imbalance.

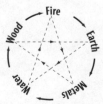

Balanced Flavors, Balanced Health

In the Chinese system, every food has one or more designated flavors, having to do with its affect on the body in addition to its actual taste. Many foods have more than one flavor, but generally one flavor is predominant. TCM recognizes five flavors: sweet, sour, bitter, pungent (or spicy), and salty. For the most part, a food's flavor is directly related to its actual taste. Lemon is sour; dandelion greens are bitter; bananas and cake are sweet; chilies and radishes are pungent. On occasion, however, foods have a designated flavor that has less to do with its taste and more to do with its properties. Meat, chicken, spinach, and beans, for instance, are considered sweet in TCM. Celery and asparagus are bitter.

A traditional Chinese meal balances each of the five flavors. According to Oriental diet theory, each flavor stimulates its corresponding organ. In balance with other flavors, it perpetuates harmony, but when in excess it may lead to a pattern of imbalance associated with that element. Choosing foods from each of the five flavors not only offers gustatory appeal, it's also an important part of keeping energy, or Qi, moving from phase to phase; it harmonizes the body, sustains health, balances emotions, calms the mind, and lifts the spirit. By choosing approximately 20 percent of our food from each flavor category, each corresponding organ system is equally stimulated, and thus the body enters a state of balance.

The best-tasting—and often healthiest—foods are complements of the five flavors. Consider this salad, for instance: The sweetness of a vine-ripened tomato complements perfectly the mildly bitter flavor of crisp romaine lettuce leaves. Toss them with a rich, earthy olive oil, a touch of softly-sweet-yet-sour balsamic vinegar, the salty tang of Parmesan cheese shavings, the deep salty richness of anchovy, and the pungency of freshly minced garlic and cracked black pepper. All together these flavors make this salad an extraordinarily delicious—and healthy—dish.

The favorite dishes of each of the world's culinary traditions bring together a balance of flavors, textures, and colors to create mouthwatering pleasures. A good Italian spaghetti sauce blends sweetness and a hint of sour from simmered ripe tomatoes together with the pungency of garlic, onions, and black pepper, the bitterness of oregano and marjoram, and just the right amount of salt. A sprinkling of Parmesan cheese rounds out the dish with a hint of earthy sourness mingled with subtle sweetness and salt. From a Chinese perspective, Parmesan cheese is salty and sour as well as sweet (the culturing imparts some sour notes, salt is added to make it and some sweetness is retained from the milk, from which it, is made.) This blend of flavors is poured over tender, sweet noodles and served along with crisp bitter salad greens dressed with the sweet, sour, and pungent flavors of oil, vinegar, and seasonings, respectively.

Although not considered the healthiest of meals, one all-American favorite, the hamburger, provides a sort of balance. The perfectly grilled juicy hamburger patty (sweet), seasoned with a sprinkling of salt and pungent ground pepper, is sandwiched between two sweet buns and dressed with the pungency of mustard and raw onion, the slight bitterness of lettuce, the cool sweetness of a slice of tomato, and the sour tartness of pickle: the American version of a balanced meal. Interestingly, the burger condiments have recently been found to impart a number of health benefits. Onions may help us digest the beef as well as reduce cholesterol levels and maintain a smooth flow of blood, reflecting the Chinese concept of the pungent flavor stimulating blood, circulation, and the heart. The tomato contains carotenoids and antioxidants which prevent the oxidation of cholesterol and its accumulation on artery walls. Ketchup, in particular, is packed with lycopene, the plant pigment associated with reduced risk of heart disease and prostate cancer. If you cut the bread and beef by half and tripled the condiments, you'd have a fairly healthy meal.

But an imbalance or excess of any one flavor can leave us suffering from various types of illnesses or discomforts. Too much or too little of any of the flavors is said to imbalance its corresponding organs, or the organ that the flavor "travels to." Each flavor can be used in greater or lesser amounts to balance a health condition or environmental situation. A steaming cup of slightly bitter coffee registers a certain quality of pleasure with your tongue and simultaneously stimulates the heart and, for a short time, liberates and moves our Qi, giving us a temporary boost of energy. But caffeinated coffee also leads to a loss of Qi, through its diuretic action and strain on the kidney system, ultimately leaving us fatigued. Sweet flavors from grains, dairy, and sugary treats—foods we tend to overuse in Western countries—most affect the spleen (the term for digestion in Chinese medicine) and the flesh. The right amount of these sweet foods warms and calms us and slows digestion, leaving us relaxed and comforted, with the lingering sensation of a full belly.

However, too much of the sweet flavor leaves us lethargic, short of breath, and often overweight. In the appropriate amounts, salty foods, another Western favorite, help maintain the kidneys and bodily fluids. But salt can burden the kidneys and contribute to calcium loss and osteoporosis when overused.[21]

Having a particular flavor in your mouth may be a sign the related organ system is out of balance. For instance, a sour taste has to do with the wood element and the corresponding organ, the liver. The intense sourness of bile may actually rise to your palate from an upset liver or gallbladder. A bitter taste in your mouth has to do with the element fire and an imbalance in the corresponding organ, the heart. A lingering sweetness in your mouth indicates an imbalance with the spleen, or digestion, and the earth element. It is most likely accompanied with digestive trouble and cravings for sweets, signs of a spleen (digestion) imbalance.

Nutrition's Color Therapy

Each flavor is part of a group of associated qualities, among them color and element. The sour flavor is associated with wood, which is likewise associated with the color green. The bitter flavor corresponds with fire, which corresponds with the color red. Sweetness corresponds with earth, and thus earth colors, especially yellow and orange. The pungent flavor corresponds with metal, as well as the color white. Saltiness is associated with water, which is associated with the dark colors. However, the flavor and the color connected to a particular element do not necessarily go together. For instance, the sour flavor is associated with the wood element, as is the color green, but not all green foods are sour and not all sour foods are green.

According to TCM, each dish should be balanced not only with respect to flavor but also in regards to color. A tender, poached white fish (sweet and white) seasoned with ginger and garlic (pungent and white) is balanced when served with spears of stir-fried asparagus (bitter and green) and slices of roasted red-chili pepper (pungent and red), with black-bean sauce (sour/salty and dark) over steamed white rice (sweet and white). A small salad of romaine lettuce or julienned turnips adds an additional touch of bitter.

For optimum flavor, presentation, and healthful balance, meals should draw from a variety of colors. A balance of colors and flavors is welcomed by the eye and the palate and experienced in the body as renewed energy, a sense of calm, and ultimately good health. In Chinese cuisine the various colors and flavors of vegetables, in particular, are a vital part of the appealing harmony created at each meal. Colors and flavors in food provide an edible balance to corresponding organs of the body. Rich orange and yellow root vegetables and winter squashes provide sweet balance to the bitter quality of dark greens. Yellow and orange harmonize the spleen, the earth element. Green is associated with the liver and the wood element. The white color and pungency of turnips or horseradish (associated with the lungs) complements a beef dish (sweet flavor associated with the digestion, or spleen) in flavor and helps with the digestion of fats in beef. The spice of chilies contrasts with the cooling mildness of an eggplant or a white bean dish, foods associated with the lungs. Western science acknowledges that colorful plant foods are rich in crucial vitamins and minerals, antioxidants, and other phytochemicals that protect us against disease and aging: dark green, orange, and red foods are recognized as healthful foods, because their pigments indicate that beneficial nutrients, such as beta-carotene and lycopene, are present. Iceberg lettuce, on the other hand, is very pale and recognized to have very little nutritional value.

Each of the various colors of food, particularly fruits and vegetables, are associated with their own healing nutrients in the West and healing qualities in the East. Blueberries are one of the richest sources of anthocyanins, compounds that can prevent blood clots, improve night vision, and slow macular degeneration. In Chinese medicine, the deep color of blueberries mean they are extremely cooling and thus beneficial to those with a pattern of heat, revealed by signs such as heart disease (clotting blood) and perhaps trouble with vision. Red pigments in tomatoes, called lycopene, and others called carotenoids, are associated with reduced cancer and heart disease risk. They might be used in a Chinese dish to harmonize the heart, which is associated with the element of fire.

Too often, Western meals are overly beige or white. Pasta with cream sauce leaves out the colors associated with wood (green), fire (red), water (black, brown, or dark blue), and earth (yellow or orange). Balance could be created with the addition of fresh parsley and roasted red peppers. A grilled cheese sandwich, which leaves out green, red, and dark colors, could be balanced with a side dish of asparagus plus sliced tomatoes. The standard steak-and-potatoes fare is lacking in green, yellow, and red—a tossed green salad with radishes would be a good complement to this meal. Cereal with milk leaves out the colors associated with wood, fire, earth, and water and would achieve better balance with the addition of strawberries and blueberries. Meals limited in color and flavor may taste good at first, or satisfy our hunger momentarily, but over time the imbalance caused by focusing on one or a couple of flavors and colors (such as sweetness or whiteness) may leave us feeling tired, depressed, or agitated.

Green, from the wood element, is the "master" color. It is the most healing of all colors and is the color generally most underused in the American diet. All body patterns benefit from green foods, such as broccoli, chard, spinach, watercress, collards, mustard greens, turnip greens, beet greens, asparagus, brussels sprouts, and other leafy greens. Green needs to balance the white of the metal element. Red from the fire element also helps to balance white from the metal element, while the golden hues of earth balance the darkness of the water element. In general, red, orange, or yellow (bright, yang colors) vegetables and fruits are more warming than green, blue, or purple (dark, yin colors) foods. Winter squashes, sweet potatoes, yams, parsnips, and chili peppers stimulate and warm the body more than eggplant, spinach, or cucumbers. Maintaining a balance of warming and cooling colors is particularly helpful to health. An imbalance of colors may lead to cravings for the wrong foods.

SAMPLE FOODS BY COLOR

Green Foods

avocados	kale
broccoli	lettuce
collard greens	limes
green apples	mustard greens
green beans	spinach
green peas	

Red Foods

Ahi tuna (Ahi is red in color as opposed to yellow or bluefin tuna, which are pale or white.)	red peppers
beets	strawberries
radishes	tomatoes

Yellow-Orange Foods

apricots	pumpkins
millet	sweet potatoes
oranges	winter squash
peaches	yams

White Foods

cauliflower	turkey
cucumbers	turnips
egg whites	water chestnuts
onions	white fish
rice	white potatoes

Dark Foods

black beans	coffee
blackberries	kelp
black sesame seeds	soy sauce
blueberries	

THE USES AND ABUSES OF THE FLAVORS

Sweetness and the Earth Element

The sweet flavor predominates in the Western diet. Sweetness is a warm, yang flavor. It's a build-up food; in other words, it helps us put on weight, not always a desirable thing. Thin, dry, emaciated people benefit from the "build-up" property of the sweet flavor in foods. We think of cookies, cake, and ice cream as our sweets. But the sweet category includes carrots, potatoes, yams, and other root vegetables, many grains, bread and cereals, milk, beans, and even meat, fish, poultry, and eggs. In fact, most of our diet comes from the sweet flavor. We tend to crave these sweets beyond the point of harmony. Simple, or refined, sugars briefly energize us but ultimately leave us fatigued, while complex carbohydrates such as breads tend to relax or even sedate the body. Overeating sweets in an attempt to either stimulate or relax ourselves burdens our digestion, leaving us overweight and, ironically, often more tired and anxious than ever, and craving more sweets.

Whole grains, beans, and dairy and animal products are considered "full sweets," meaning these foods are nourishing, fulfilling, and satisfying. Foods containing an abundance of simple sugars, including sweetened fruits, candy, cookies, and other treats, are "empty sweets" and can leave us unsatisfied and intensify our cravings for refined sugar-rich foods.

Full sweets, such as meats and poultry, rice, sweet potatoes, and whole grains, as well as small amounts of certain empty sweets like honey or molasses, are considered strengthening foods, beneficial for someone recovering from an illness or surgery. In appropriate amounts, full sweet foods strengthen our spleen system and immunity. In excess, any sweet foods, especially refined sweets, weaken digestion and spleen Qi, thereby weakening immunity, leaving us prone to colds and flu. In excess, they also lead to weight gain.

Appropriate quantities of sweet vegetables, whole grains, and fruits calm someone with irritability from an overheated, liver and moisten dry conditions. Such healthful sweet foods also slow down an overactive heart and mind. A "sweet" snack of baked potato, sweet rice, oatmeal, or fruit can help relax the body and induce sleep, a reflection of the sweet flavor's ability to sedate the restless "heart," according to Chinese medicine. Western biochemistry details the pathway whereby such foods stimulate the release of serotonin, a yin brain chemical associated with a sense of calm, happiness, and relaxation.

Those who most benefit from full sweets include those who are thin, dry, and nervous. Those who are restless and always worrying may find balance from shifting away from refined sugar and meats and focusing more on cooked vegetables, fish, beans, and whole grains. Sweets should be used sparingly by those who are overweight and often lethargic and tired—for these people, in particular, too many breads, grains, and refined sweets may lead to excess weight gain, digestive problems (including bloating), sugar cravings, fatigue, anxiety, water retention, mucous production, and weakened bones. Sweet foods are healthful and don't lead to such problems when balanced with bitter, pungent, and sour flavors.

FULL SWEET FOODS

apricots	grapes
barley	kamut
beans	lentils
beef	milk
beets	millet
carrots	nuts
chard	olives
cherries	parsnips
cheese*,**	peas
chicken	pork
corn	potatoes
dates	rice
eggplant	spelt
eggs	spinach
fish	wheat
figs	yogurt**
grapes	

EMPTY SWEET FOODS

barley-malt syrup	maple syrup
fructose	molasses
fruit-juice sweeteners	rice syrup
honey	white sugar (sucrose)

*also salty
**also sour

Bitterness and the Fire Element

The bitter flavor in Chinese medicine is yin and generally considered the most cooling and drying of the flavors. It is one of the most underused flavors in American cooking. Bitterness contracts our energy, drawing it inward. It is thus purging and helps balance overweight, abdominal bloating and distention, gas, and water retention as well as irritability, a heated temper, red acne, and herpes. Bitter foods, especially greens and rye, are among the most beneficial foods for weight loss. Those who benefit most from the addition of greens and other bitter foods are those who tend toward being overweight, who feel hot most of the time, who are loud spoken and talkative, and who have high blood pressure, a red complexion, and frequent headaches.

Bitter is the healing flavor for the heart and the antidote for a hot climate, or summer, the associated season. Its cooling nature sedates fire, the corresponding element. Lettuces, alfalfa sprouts, asparagus, arugula, and other bitter greens are cooling foods for summer. Occasionally, bitter foods can be warming, as is the case with garlic and leeks.

People in Asian and European countries often use bitters to help with digestion and reduce risk of infection by parasites. A common European herbal remedy, "digestive bitters" are taken before meals to stimulate flow of digestive juices, increase the strength of peristaltic waves, and promote the effective mixing and moving of food.[22] Bitter foods and herbs have antibiotic properties and are helpful in destroying parasites. The spicy, bitter, green Japanese condiment, wasabe, served with sushi, is thought to minimize the risk of parasites from raw fish.

Bitter foods are also anti-inflammatory. A diet abundant in bitter greens helps reduce joint pain in those with rheumatism. The bitter flavor helps keep the arteries clear of cholesterol and fats. Bitter foods such as greens, green tea, and garlic have been shown through studies to reduce cholesterol levels and keep blood flowing smoothly. Greens and rye are also rich in magnesium, a nutrient critical for heart function and often lacking in the American diet. Greens are also a good source of carotenoids, which are essential for artery and heart health, and iron, which is important for building blood.

Bitter-tasting foods can help offset the effects of stress and overuse of alcohol on the liver. Too much work, too many deadlines or frustrations in life, as well as overuse of alcohol or drugs (medical or otherwise) overburden the liver, congesting energy or Qi, which leads to the buildup of heat in this organ system. When there is heat in the liver, restlessness mounts, tempers flare, and impatience interferes with harmonious relationships. The bitter flavor is said to clear heat, or fire, from the liver. In Western medical terms, greens contain antioxidants and liver-detoxifying nutrients and enzymes, which help the liver deal with burdens of stress hormones and toxins. The cooling nature of bitter greens such as romaine lettuce, dandelion leaves, or watercress sedates and calms an overheated liver, mellowing a tendency toward anger, impatience, and agitation.

Coffee and chocolate are among the most popular bitter-flavored foods in Western societies. I often suspect that cravings for chocolate and coffee may be our desire for more of the bitter flavor in our diet. Unfortunately, chocolate is made palatable by the addition of copious amounts of sugar and cream, two substances that contribute to such problems as obesity, fatigue, and indigestion. While some coffee stimulates the heart and the digestive system, too much coffee overstimulates the heart and weakens the kidneys, leading to fatigue, weakened bones, nervousness, and sometimes digestive problems.

Overuse of the bitter flavor can lead to diarrhea and dehydration, and can dry and wither the skin. The bitter flavor should be used judiciously by those who are cold, weak, thin, nervous, and dry skinned. To minimize the dehydrating, withering effect of bitter foods, they are best combined with sweet or salty foods. It is interesting we enjoy the bitter quality of coffee softened with the moistening sweetness of milk, cream, or sugar. Rye is the bread of choice for a sandwich of sweet and salty corned beef. Romaine lettuce is sumptuously complemented with the sweet-salty-sour flavor of Parmesan cheese in a Caesar salad.

BITTER FOODS

alfalfa sprouts*	rye
arugula*	pumpkin seeds*
asparagus**	kohlrabi**,***
broccoli***	radish leaves
broccoli rabe***	marjoram
celery*	oregano
collard greens	scallions***
dandelion greens*	turnips**,***
kale**,***	vinegar****
lettuce**	watercress***
romaine lettuce	white pepper***

*also salty
**also sweet
***also pungent
****also sour

Sour and the Wood Element

The sour flavor of a lemon, grapefruit, or a tart young apple is yin and cooling. It is associated the liver function, the color green, and spring, when plants are young and immature. Many of the tender spring greens and early berries taste sour and have yet to achieve the full sweetness of fruits in summer. Sourness demands balance from sweetness; we relish sour foods sweetened with sugar, such as cranberry sauce, lemon custard, lemonade, and rhubarb pie.

The sour flavor can help an overactive liver. "Sour substances are astringent and prevent or reverse the abnormal leakage of fluids and energy," says the *Nei Jing Huandgdi's Internal Classic* by the Yellow Emperor, a famous healer during the Han dynasty. The puckering quality of the sour flavor makes it useful in the treatment of urinary incontinence, excessive perspiration, diarrhea, and sagging tissues. The acidity of sour foods facilitates the release of saliva and hydrochloric acid in the stomach, enhancing digestion.

The sour flavor is cleansing, enabling fat-soluble toxins to become more water-soluble and better excreted by the kidneys.[23] It is thought to counteract the effects of rich, greasy food. In Western nutrition, we incorporate lemon and grapefruit into liver-cleansing programs. The use of sour foods in a liver-cleanse helps to cool the agitation and anger associated with an overworked, stressed liver.

Too much sour flavor, however, overstimulates the liver, as well as the tendons. An overstimulated liver is said to "invade" the spleen, interfering with digestion and appetite. Too much of the sour favor leads to dampness and thus can impair the normal flow of Qi, or energy. Bloating, fatigue, and cravings for sweets (the balance flavor to sour) may result. Excess sour flavor also weakens the muscles and may aggravate rheumatism. It also may harden and wrinkle the skin, causing the lips to become dry and cracked. Those with constipation or dampness should go light on the sour flavor. The excesses or problems brought on by too much sour flavor can be relieved by the pungent, Qi-stimulating flavor of foods such as turnips, radishes, hot peppers, and black pepper.

SOUR FOODS

adzuki beans**
apples**
blackberries**
cheese*
crabapples**
cranberries**
currants**
citrus fruits
grapes**
grapefruit**
huckleberries**
leeks

miso soup*
oranges**
pickles*
plums**
raspberries**
sauerkraut
strawberries**
tangerines**
tomatoes**
vinegar**
yogurt**

*also salty
**also sweet

Saltiness and the Water Element

The salty flavor of well-seasoned soups and sauces, soy sauce, condiments, and the white crystals pressed into your favorite pretzels is generally yin, cooling, and moistening. Salt is associated with the kidney function, the element water, and the winter season. Sea vegetables—plants rich in salt, magnesium, and calcium—are particularly cooling and moistening and provide nutrients and therapeutic value to those at risk of heart disease and with high blood pressure. However, salty foods can be warming when used in excess, especially in the form of French fries, potato chips, fried meats, or other greasy, salty foods.

Along with the overuse of sugar, the Western diet is generally too salty. Salt shakers sit at every eating space, and processed foods and snacks are packed with over-processed salt, which leaves a higher concentration of sodium chloride than a less-processed, natural version of salt (often sold as "sea salt"). Excess salt, in many people, contributes to high blood pressure, water retention, and an imbalance of other minerals, including potassium, magnesium, and calcium. It is also a dietary culprit in weakening bones. Interestingly, in TCM, too much salt is said to harm the bones and blood.

Overindulging in salty foods often leads to cravings for sweets, leading to a vicious cycle of alternating sugar and salt cravings.

That said, some salt is necessary for normal kidney function and the maintenance of fluids and warmth in the body. Occasionally I see a client who is not getting enough salt. Low energy, a pale complexion, dizziness upon standing, and low blood pressure are signs that there may not be enough salt in the diet.

Emily came to me for nutrition counseling because she was exhausted and fatigued, had dark circles under her eyes, was often cold, and tended to feel depressed. She often felt lightheaded, especially when she stood up too quickly. When I asked about her diet, she said it was very healthy. Ever since her husband had been diagnosed with heart disease over a year ago, their meals had been strictly vegetarian with no added salt. Emily had been living on a nearly salt-free diet, and she was actually salt-deficient. Shortly after the addition of small amounts of salt to her diet, her flagging energy picked up, she feel more energized, the dark circles faded, and she warmed up.

The Chinese salt of choice is not from the salt shaker, but rather from soy sauce and sea vegetables. Seaweed, or sea vegetables, are a rich source of magnesium, potassium, calcium, protein, and even essential fats. Sea vegetables are used in Chinese culinary medicine to soften hard masses, including stones and tumors. They contribute the minerals that help build bones and calm emotions.

The best salt choices include sea salt, soy sauce, and shoyu or tamari sauces (types of soy sauce), as opposed to highly processed table salt. Sea salt provides other trace minerals important to balance in the body. Parsley and celery are plant foods that have a salty flavor.

SALTY FOODS

alfalfa sprouts*	sea salt
arugula*	sea vegetables
celery*	shoyu sauce
dandelion leaves*	soy sauce
parsley*	
tamari sauce	

*also bitter

Pungency and the Metal Element

The subtle bite of turnips and horseradish and the stimulating warmth of spicy chilies and garlic are yang, warming qualities characteristic of most pungent foods. The pungent flavor brings energy from the core of the body outward, dispersing poor circulation. It is associated with the autumn season, the element metal, and the color white. The corresponding environmental influence is dryness. In Chinese medicine, the pungent flavor of herbs and foods are used to disperse or dry congestion, especially respiratory infections. In balanced amounts, pungent foods help keep the lungs clear and open.

Warming pungent foods, such as mustard seeds, garlic, cumin, and cayenne, help stimulate a sluggish or slow digestion. Cooling pungent foods, including peppermint tea and radishes, daikon root, and marjoram, are helpful when high blood pressure is coupled with high cholesterol levels, overweight, and anger or irritability.

The pungent flavor moves life energy, or Qi, warming and stimulating the body. Those who feel cold, withdrawn, and depressed much of the time benefit from the warming, expansive nature of pungent foods. The pungent flavor nourishes the lungs, dispersing phlegm and mucous. Spicy foods increase the flow of blood, warming various organs and stimulating metabolic activity throughout the body. The mucous-clearing effect of pungent herbs and foods can also benefit digestion and the urinary tract. Therapeutic uses for the pungent flavor include stimulating a slow metabolism, improving digestion, clearing mucous, and relieving arthritis.[24]

The spiciness of chilies, while adding a piquant flavor to a stir-fried beef dish, also facilitates digestion of the beef by stimulating gastric secretions to break down protein. Though chilies are initially warming (and are thereby considered a yang food in Chinese medicine), their ability to promote perspiration ultimately cools the body, providing a cooling balance to the warming nature of beef. They can also cool the body in hot weather. Appropriately, chilies grow and tend to be popular in hot climates, including southern China and Latin America.

Too many pungent foods, which stimulate bursts of energy movement, are said to exhaust our Qi. The associated tissue of the metal element is skin and hair. With an excess of pungent or spicy foods, skin and hair may become dry. The drying action can lead to constipation or a dry cough. Too much black pepper, garlic, cayenne, raw onion, peppermint tea, or other pungent-flavored foods can dry the lungs, skin, digestion, and mucous membranes, leading to imbalance.

WARMING PUNGENT FOODS

anise seed

basil**,****

black pepper

broccoli rabe***

cabbage**

cayenne

celery seed

chilies

cinnamon

cloves

cumin seed

fennel seed

garlic and other onion family members

ginger

horseradish

kale**,***

leeks****

mustard greens

mustard seed

nutmeg*

oregano

parsley*,***

rosemary

spearmint

turmeric***

watercress***

COOLING OR NEUTRAL PUNGENT FOODS

broccoli***

celery

daikon

kohlrabi**,***

marjoram**,***

oregano**,***

peppermint

radishes

turnips**,***

watercress***

white pepper

*also salty

**also sweet

***also bitter

****also sour

Learning from Flavor Cravings

When in balance, we are naturally drawn to foods that will maintain that balance and nourish us on every level. If we become out of whack either physically or emotionally, we start to crave certain foods to restore balance. Usually our bodies tell us exactly what we need: Someone who is chilled and anemic may long for a steak, while someone who's been playing basketball on a summer afternoon relishes a slice of watermelon. However, sometimes we crave foods (particularly sweet and salty ones) that bring a temporary feeling of balance but ultimately weaken and further imbalance us.

The week before her period starts, Cindy craves all things chocolate. "I'll eat chocolate ice cream, milk- or dark-chocolate candies, or handfuls of chocolate chips, if they're in front of me," says Cindy. Women frequently crave breads, pasta, cookies, cake, candy, muffins, and other sweets. The cause of a craving can often be determined by understanding the Five Element Cycle and the nature of the elements.

Cravings for chocolate, a bitter, cooling flavor, may be an attempt to quench the hot, yang state of the body (in particular, the liver) characteristic of PMS for many women. The sugary component of most chocolate foods is temporarily calming to the nerves. A healthy alternative is to regularly consume bitter leafy greens, including arugula, romaine lettuce, broccoli, dandelion greens, asparagus, and turnip and mustard greens. Bitter greens keep the liver calm and soothed and thus premenstrual tension at bay. Greens are a good source of magnesium and folic acid, nutrients needed to make serotonin, a brain chemical that induces calm and controls carbohydrate cravings.

The craving for a particular flavor may indicate an imbalance in the corresponding organ. Sugar cravings, which often accompany fatigue, are a sign that the spleen/stomach (digestion process) is out of balance. The spleen corresponds with the earth element and the sweet flavor. One way the spleen becomes weakened is through a diet lacking in protein from beef, pork, poultry, seafood, or eggs. The result is often cravings for concentrated refined sweets, such as cookies and candy, in order to derive enough of the qualities of the earth element, associated with the sweet flavor. Once you start enjoying the intense sweetness of things like cookies, sodas, and candy, resisting them becomes increasingly difficult. Eating too many of these sugary foods further weakens spleen function, leading to increasing problems with digestion, fatigue, and cravings for more sugar to boost flagging energy levels. Here, an imbalance strives to perpetuate itself through increasing cravings for more sugar.

Vegetarians with sugar cravings and low energy are often suffering from weak spleen Qi and may find relief by adding eggs or fish to their diet. Another option for vegetarians who want to stay that way is to eat plenty of well-cooked, well-chewed grains, lots of cooked vegetables, warming seasonings, as well as beans, peas, lentils, and other protein sources to build spleen Qi (or digestion), described in chapter three.

As with sugar, our palates can become accustomed to increasing amounts of salt. A craving for salty snack foods and a heavy hand with the salt shaker may indicate trouble in the kidneys and a cold pattern of imbalance. The kidneys are associated with the water element and salty flavor. Signs of kidney weakness may include low back or knee pain, cold hands and feet, and dark circles under the eyes. Including adequate salt is important, but too much weakens the kidneys and their function. Slowly reducing salty foods and use of salt allows the palate to adjust to less salt.

Overeating sweets can set you up to want excess salt. The reverse is also true. By overeating the water element flavor, or salt, you may wind up with cravings for the earth element flavor, sweetness, for balance.

---

21. Silver, J., et al., "Sodium-dependent idiopathic hypercalciura in renal-stone formers," *Lancet* 2 (1983): 484–86.
22. Tierra, Michael, C.A.,N.D., *Planetary Herbology*, Santa Fe: Lotus Press, (1988): 410.
23. Ibid., 409.
24. Ibid., 34.

3

STRONG SPLEEN QI:
OPTIMIZING HEALTH AND WEIGHT
THROUGH BALANCED DIGESTION

Good digestion is the foundation of optimum health, ideal weight, mental clarity, sustained energy, and balanced moods. No matter how much you eat, if your digestive system can't properly break down and absorb nourishment from your food, you are essentially starving your body, mind, and spirit. Although both Eastern and Western health authorities believe that good digestion plays a role in overall health, they diverge in their particular perspectives on how digestion works, how it affects the body and mind, and how it responds to particular foods.

Western science looks at digestion as a measurable process of mechanical and chemical reactions, starting in the mouth and ending at the large intestine, with the critical processes occurring in the gut—the stomach, pancreas, liver and bile, the intestines, and the colon. If you don't have heartburn, acid reflux, excess gas, constipation, diarrhea, or undigested food in your stools, your digestion is thought to be in working order. If you do suffer from symptoms of indigestion, laxatives, antacids, and a variety of other modern drugs are readily available. However, many of the discomforts associated with eating and digesting are not resolved through Western treatments and may even be made worse by these drugs. Laxatives, for instance, may become addictive. Antacids are often prescribed when the problem is lack of stomach acid, not too much.

The Chinese view digestion more holistically, as influenced by the particular foods we eat, our states of mind, and the health of our organs. TCM gives specific meaning to all the subtle and not-so-subtle irritations we experience when things having to do with eating, assimilating, or eliminating food aren't quite right: the lingering feeling of fullness long after a meal or even a snack, a frequent craving for sugar, sluggish elimination, loose stools, a dry mouth and throat, a burning sensation in the stomach between meals, bloating after eating, and even fatigue. Instead of using drugs to alleviate symptoms, Chinese medicine emphasizes specific foods and restricts others to balance the organs contributing to signs of discomfort.

According to TCM, good digestion requires appropriate food choices for one's individual body pattern. As you will learn in the next chapter, each of us differs in our physical needs as well as in our mental and emotional tendencies; accordingly, we each respond differently to foods. For example, although they are considered healthful by Western nutrition standards, salads and whole wheat bread aren't appropriate for all digestive systems. From a TCM standpoint, fresh fruit actually may be a bad choice in certain situations. Even those foods we grew up thinking were good for us can in fact lead to digestive and other health problems if we are unable to assimilate them optimally.

THE BUBBLING CAULDRON:
DIGESTION FROM THE CHINESE PERSPECTIVE

Famous for their use of metaphor and pictures depicting life, the Chinese view digestion as a bubbling cauldron with a hot flame (called *digestive fire*) burning beneath it. When digestive fire is strong and the mix in the pot is balanced—just the right pungency, sweetness, and salt, the right level of moisture, the right temperature—digestion proceeds smoothly, and food is effectively converted to fuel. Under these optimal conditions, your appetite is good and your meals provide satisfaction. After eating, you have a subtle feeling of movement in the belly as this bubbling pot transforms your food into life-giving energy and directs it throughout the body. When digestion is healthy and the organs are in balance, your mind and body are suffused with a vitality that catalyzes new thoughts and ideas and gives you the fortitude to bring projects to completion.

Chinese medicine refers to the collection of organs and tissues that digest or transform our food into body tissue, warmth, and energy as the *spleen*, or sometimes as the *spleen/pancreas* for clarity, since the pancreas is the organ that releases most of the hormones and enzymes involved in digestion. The Chinese concept of spleen has almost nothing to do with the organ of the same name in Western physiology. In the Western view, the spleen plays a role in immunity as well as in storing and releasing blood. In TCM, this organ is considered more like a second liver, and the term *spleen* refers not so much to a distinct organ or tissue as to a system which includes the digestive functions of the liver, gallbladder, and pancreas, as well as their hormones, enzymes, acids, and other secretions. Throughout this book, the term signifies the Chinese process of digestion rather than the relatively minor organ described in Western physiology.

The spleen's partner, the stomach, serves as the cauldron that receives our food. The spleen acts like a flame and distillation system: The heat of the flame transforms the chewed mix in the stomach into a bubbling, fermenting soup. The resulting energy, or Qi, is said to rise from the digestive area to the lungs, where it joins with Qi from air, giving us breath. The purified liquids from digestion are separated and rise to the heart, where they form blood. The stomach helps separate out waste and moves it downward for elimination.

Food-Qi, or the vital energy we get from food, is the Chinese equivalent of adenosine triphosphate (ATP), the energy the body uses for warmth and all physical activity. Just like ATP, Qi gives us energy. Here, however, the similarities between the two concepts end. "The concept of Qi is absolutely at the heart of Chinese medicine," say Harriet Beinfield and Efrem Korngold, authors of the Chinese medicine classic *Between Heaven and Earth.*[25] Qi is said to permeate all living and non-living things. Qi gives rise to life. It is energy becoming matter, and it can perpetuate itself. ATP is generated by specific biochemical reactions in the body; it can be isolated, observed, and quantified. Qi, on the other hand, can be known or experienced only through its effects.

A healthy flow of Qi is critical to good digestion. If Qi becomes blocked in an organ or moves in the wrong direction, health problems arise. Attaining optimum digestion (called *strong spleen Qi* in TCM) requires the creation of an ideal "soup-like" mixture in the stomach and maintaining the strong, steady flame of the spleen. The key to both of these desired states is a balance of moisture and dryness as well as optimum temperature. We often eat and behave in ways that create excessive dampness, dryness, cold, or heat, all of which can disrupt Qi, leaving us with indigestion, bloating, stomach ulcers, low energy, food cravings, and weight problems.

The stomach itself needs to maintain a certain degree of moistness and a moderate temperature (including adequate mucous and digestive secretions and just the right amount of stomach acid, in Western terms) in order to properly ferment its contents. Moisture and temperature, after all, are important in other types of fermentation, from composting to wine making. In TCM, the stomach is said to "like moisture" and "dislike dryness." The depletion of stomach fluids, sometimes called *stomach-yin deficiency* (fluids are yin), can result from skipped meals, irregular eating patterns, worrying or working while eating, consuming too many fried foods or poor quality fats, and particularly eating late at night. Signs of stomach-yin deficiency include feeling uncomfortably warm in the afternoons, a dry mouth and throat with little true thirst, and dry stools, perhaps with constipation.

Even more troublesome than stomach-yin deficiency is *stomach fire*, a condition brought on by mental stress and overwork, as well as overeating, heating substances such as alcohol, spicy foods, fried foods, poor quality vegetable oils (partially hydrogenated vegetable oils, heat processed, overheated or old oils), red meat, coffee, and citrus fruits. This condition is characterized by a burning sensation in the stomach, stomach ulcers, bleeding gums, canker sores, a voracious appetite, bad breath, and constipation.

The spleen, on the other hand, is especially sensitive to moisture and functions best when kept from becoming "damp," which makes sense when you view the spleen as a flame: Too much moisture can dampen the flame, which facilitates the ripening of the food mass and the distillation system that separates out the usable parts of our food. When digestive fire is strong, the spleen can readily fulfill its distillation role and separate the "pure" from the "impure" parts of our food. Healthy digestive fire, then, is maintained by choosing foods and following eating patterns that keep the flame burning consistently.

In TCM, a damp spleen can lead to the well-known Western problems of obesity, parasites (including yeast overgrowth), cysts, tumors, abdominal bloating, water retention, and a general feeling of heaviness. Habits that contribute to a damp spleen include consuming too many cold foods (iced water and sodas, frozen desserts, smoothies), dairy products, raw fruits, juices, and salads, as well as living in an overly damp or moldy environment.

THE BENEFITS OF GOOD DIGESTION OR STRONG SPLEEN QI

From a Western perspective, healthy digestion means no more gas, heartburn, or constipation. TCM, on the other hand, gives much greater significance to the role of spleen Qi. When the spleen is balanced and spleen Qi is strong, not only do we enjoy optimum health, strength, and vitality, but we are also better able to manifest our ideas and goals. Strong spleen Qi enables us to more easily accomplish tasks, be it writing a report or sewing a quilt. Strong spleen Qi gets skyscrapers and bridges erected, superhighways constructed, and cities built. Healthy spleen Qi is something you can feel throughout your body. It's the mental and physical energy that drives you to finish a project.

A strong spleen is experienced specifically in the muscles of your legs and arms. Poor spleen Qi leaves the limbs feeling weak. Strong spleen Qi is the strength and fortitude that course through your thighs as you push down on the pedals of your bicycle to carry you up a hill. Good spleen Qi provides the determination and strength it takes to clean out the garage: lifting, dragging, and reorganizing boxes, bags, and tools and throwing out debris. It takes good spleen Qi to build a fence, to plant a garden, and to bake a cake. Martha Stewart has good spleen Qi.

Healthy spleen Qi also nourishes the mind, providing mental strength and the ability to concentrate and focus. It takes good spleen Qi to keep your files and desk orderly, to balance your checkbook, to create a marketing plan, and to study for an exam. Strong spleen Qi enables us to focus, to concentrate, and to recall information. You can't memorize difficult exam material without a strong spleen.

Strong spleen Qi, as you will learn, requires regular, nourishing meals. Getting adequate meat and complex carbohydrates, in particular, build strong spleen Qi. The widespread meat and potato fare, once the standard among Americans, coincided with the greatest period of building and expansion in our history. America was built on an abundance of spleen Qi. On the other hand, the impoverished living conditions in some third-world countries reflect the inhabitants' weak spleen Qi as a result lack of food, and in particular lack of protein. Inadequate food and the lack of animal products, especially, in the diet weaken spleen Qi.

What this all means is that strong, healthy spleen Qi—otherwise known as good digestion—converts our food into high-quality mental and physical energy, vitality, and good health. Although the concept of Qi, or vital energy, coursing throughout the body and mind and making us productive is foreign to the Western way of thinking, it provides a practical model for working with Chinese nutrition, acupuncture, and other therapies. The right food choices for your type should leave you satisfied and comfortable after eating. They should promote mental and physical energy and stamina, as well as strength and tone in the arms and legs. When digestion is healthy, according to Chinese medicine, the mind is clear and focused, and we are productive and responsible in our lives.

SIGNS OF STRONG SPLEEN QI/GOOD DIGESTION

daily, complete elimination (bowel movements)
feeling good after elimination
feeling alert and clear headed after eating
pleasant taste in mouth
normal body weight
good muscle tone
able to work hard
practical and responsible
strong, active, stable
good endurance
healthy appetite and satisfaction after meals

HOW WE END UP WITH POOR DIGESTION
AND EXCESS WEIGHT GAIN

We sometimes lose sight of the purpose and tremendous power of food. We eat just to fill our stomach or to take away hunger. We often choose foods not so much because they are good for us but because they seem appealing: a smooth, cool chocolate shake, a warm cinnamon roll, a juicy, flame-broiled burger. We drink coffee or eat chocolate for energy. We eat a half a loaf of warm buttered bread to quell the pain of loneliness. We crunch through potato chips to distract us from anxiety. We grab handfuls of nuts and wash them down with icy cold sodas or beer while engrossed in a football game or at a party. More often than not, these choices give us indigestion, weakening our spleen Qi, and leaving us feeling tired, bloated, and lethargic and wanting more of these health-eroding foods for relief, like smokers who crave cigarettes.

There's no mistaking the results of these poor eating habits: abdominal bloating, gas, heartburn, gastric ulcers, stomach pains, constipation or diarrhea, and changes in weight and appetite. Any one of these symptoms can ruin your day. But when your digestion isn't at its best, you also can't absorb nutrients from your food, and your brain can't make the neurochemicals that keep you happy, relaxed, and focused. Poor digestion can lead to depression. Immunity suffers because inadequate nutrients reach the blood stream. Infection and disease take hold more easily. When food isn't effectively converted into energy, we don't feel energized or motivated. We lose muscle tone because our muscles don't receive amino acids for their growth and maintenance. According to TCM, these are the signs of weak spleen Qi.

SIGNS OF SPLEEN QI DEFICIENCY

loose stool or constipation

discomfort in intestines and stomach

abdominal bloating, gas

burping, heartburn

headache

nausea

too much or too little appetite

fuzzy-headed after eating

cravings for stimulants, fats, and cold,
    spicy, salty, or sweet foods

sweet or bitter taste in mouth

over- or underweight

weak arms and legs

inability to build muscle

dry, pale, or chapped lips

sallow complexion

skin eruptions

prolapsed organs (uterus, anus, stomach)

fatigue, weakness, or tiredness

depression, irritability

mental stagnation, feeling "stuck"

Poor digestion in Western terms is essentially the same thing as a stomach or spleen imbalance in TCM. Irregular eating patterns, poor food choices, and excessive mental effort or worry can lead to *stomach-yin deficiency, stomach fire,* or *spleen Qi deficiency.* Spleen Qi deficiency is the most common cause of digestive ailments in Western populations. Certain American eating habits and food choices can cause spleen Qi deficiency to give rise to a pattern of imbalance called *dampness* in the spleen.

Dampness is often accompanied by loose stool, bloating, abdominal distension, poor appetite, and irritable bowel symptoms, as well as weakness and fatigue. More progressive Western nutritionists have identified many of these digestive problems as food sensitivities, or food allergies. The offending foods are often damp-producing (dairy, wheat, sugar), according to Chinese medicine. Once spleen health is restored, many "food sensitivities" are resolved.

Dampness can be accompanied by a pattern of cold, which results from taking in too many cold foods, including cold drinks and frozen desserts as well as salads, raw fruits, and juices. Symptoms include watery stool, slow metabolism with difficulty losing weight, and a particular sensitivity to cold weather. A cold pattern is likely to leave us pale and chilled, with cold hands and feet. Dampness can also be accompanied by a pattern of heat, resulting from eating too many damp- and heat-producing foods, such as refined sweets, fatty meats, and greasy foods. Symptoms may include foul-smelling stool and gas, abdominal bloating, nausea, hemorrhoids, a burning sensation at the anus, and dark urine.

The spleen's role is to transform fluids in the digestive system, converting them into energy, movement, breath, and blood. If a spleen imbalance is allowed to persist, dampness can spread to other parts of the body, creating chronic problems. Dampness leaves you feeling heavy, unmotivated, and tired, as if you had bags of water strapped to your legs and arms. It can show up as fluids that collect in the tissues of the face, ankles, legs, or stomach, or as mucous or phlegm in the sinus, vagina, or digestive tract. Spring hay fever is dampness. So is a mucous-producing head cold. Vaginal infections, such as yeast, and inflammation in the intestines with mucous in the stool are signs of dampness. Dampness can take the form of mucous deposits or moist accumulations such as cysts and tumors. Parasites, including the over growth of harmful bacteria, are associated with damp conditions; they thrive in dampness and perpetuate it. Food poisoning, with symptoms of infection, foul-smelling gas, abdominal bloating, and diarrhea, is an example of dampness with heat. The spleen's ability to transform food into Qi is thwarted by dampness, causing a sense of fatigue, especially with a feeling of heaviness in the head, something like "brain fog."

Excess body fat is also damp. The fatty bulges that accumulate around your hips, thighs, and belly is dampness. Dampness can lead to a vicious cycle of lethargy, lack of motivation to exercise, and a spiraling weight-gain problem. It's difficult to motivate yourself to exercise if you are carrying around ten, twenty, or a hundred extra pounds of weight or if your belly is bloated with fluid. From a Chinese perspective, a strong, balanced spleen keeps digestive fire up, transforming food and beverages into energy before they become dampness and thus keeping excess fat from being stored. (See chapter eight for a more in-depth discussion of damp patterns.)

SIGNS OF DAMPNESS IN THE SPLEEN

loose stool, diarrhea	sweet taste in the mouth
foul-smelling stool	thirst with no desire to drink
abdominal bloating	food allergies
lack of appetite, a feeling of fullness	

SIGNS OF DAMPNESS SPREADING TO THE BODY

heaviness in the lower body and limbs	difficulty losing weight
fogginess in the head, dull headache	fatigue, lethargy
stuffiness in the chest	strong dislike of damp environments and humidity
mucous production in the sinuses	tumors, cysts, masses
water retention	

COMMON CAUSES OF WEAK SPLEEN QI

Digestion, and therefore spleen and stomach health, can be influenced by a number of factors, including food choices, eating habits, environmental conditions, and emotional states. Certain medications, including aspirin and other pain killers, antibiotics, cholesterol-lowering drugs, and antacids, can also weaken digestion. We often develop reactions or signs of imbalance to certain foods that we eat daily and year-round. These foods tend to be particularly heating, cooling, or damp and often include wheat products (bread, pasta, and so on), dairy products, citrus fruits, coffee, alcohol, tomatoes, potatoes, and eggs. The following are the most common causes of poor digestion, or unbalanced spleen.

Too Many Cold and Damp Foods and Beverages

Jackie, a thirty-one-year old stay-at-home mom, came to me complaining of weight gain, water retention, and fatigue. Her face was pale and puffy. She said despite regular exercise with her personal trainer, her muscles lacked tone. Although bundled in several layers, Jackie said she was cold and felt that way much of the time. Jackie had signs of cold and dampness. Her diet was a big part of the problem.

Jackie's typical breakfast was a smoothie of frozen berries, ice, protein powder, and non-fat milk. For lunch, it was salads or yogurt (sometimes a frozen yogurt) with iced tea. Dinners were often pasta with raw vegetables, salads, tofu dishes, or, when rushed, a Slim-Fast™. She frequently snacked on frozen yogurt and sipped on iced diet sodas.

The spleen likes to be warm and dry, according to Chinese medical texts. Unfortunately, Americans often mistakenly take nutritional recommendations to an extreme, believing that if some raw fruits and vegetables, tofu, and other "healthy" foods are good, a lot must be better. However, eating too many raw fruits, salads, tofu, and dairy products, as well as drinking too many juices and iced water, for prolonged periods or in the wrong type of individual, can lead to weak spleen Qi, digestive problems, and dampness. Once the spleen becomes damp, other parts of the body more readily retain fat, fluids, mucous, and masses.

The common American practice of drinking iced water, icy sodas, cold beers, and juices and of eating ice cream and frozen yogurt weaken digestive fire, the flame that transforms food into fuel and energy. A regular diet of such cold foods extinguishes digestive fire and leads to dampness and a host of health problems.

In addition to foods that are cold in temperature, *energetically* cold foods can also contribute to signs of dampness and cold. This concept has little to do with physical temperature—some foods impart cold and dampness to the body despite being served at room temperature or even warm. Salads, raw fruits and vegetables, juices, dairy products, and tofu are examples of cooling, damp foods. Cold juices, frozen yogurt, ice cream, and chilled fruits are particularly cold because they combine energetic coolness with their cold temperature. White-flour products, including white bread, most pasta, refined sweetened breakfast cereals, bagels, and crackers often lead to bloating and gas, signs of their damp and slightly cooling nature. In excess, any of these foods can lead to imbalance.

If you have frequent gas, bloating, and loose stools, or if you crave sugar, you may find relief by reducing salads and raw vegetables and replacing them with cooked vegetables and grains, legumes, meat, poultry, and fish. On the other hand, if you tend to be hot much of the time, have a red or ruddy face, a tendency toward irritability, or a heated temper and high blood pressure, you may find raw vegetables and fruits actually help you to feel better. (See chapter six for more on a heat pattern).

Too Much Refined Sugar

Tom, a forty-eight-year-old stockbroker, craves sweets. On a typical day, in addition to three hearty meals, this ruddy-faced and restless heavyset man devours two sweet rolls, drinks two or three sodas, eats a few handfuls of cookies, and often downs several hard candies. His weight is twenty pounds over his ideal and his blood pressure is elevated. He suffers from heartburn, gas, stomach ulcers, and abdominal bloating. Tom tends to get agitated yet also often feels "spacey" and forgetful. He has signs of dampness and heat.

Candy, cookies, cake, sodas, and other sources of refined sugars, such as sucrose, fructose, corn syrup, honey, concentrated fruit juice, and syrups, promote dampness when consumed in excess. Because they tend to be warming as well as damp-producing, they can lead to signs of dampness and heat. White and brown sugars are the worst culprits, since they are more concentrated than other sweeteners.

In TCM, small amounts of sweet foods are considered beneficial in moistening and warming the body. Too many cookies, candy, and other sweets, however, can create an imbalance, resulting in excess weight gain and conditions such as vaginal yeast infections, hemorrhoids, irritable bowel symptoms, acne, headaches, sinus problems, fluid retention, bloating, mood swings, fatigue, and forgetfulness, as well as high triglycerides and elevated blood pressure. In fact, a number of doctors target sugar consumption as a greater contributor to obesity, heart disease, and cancer than fat intake.[26] One's body pattern has a lot to do with how sugar and refined flours are assimilated. For individuals with patterns of dampness, sugar may be more of a health hazard than for those with other patterns.

Eating Too Fast, Too Much, or Too Late

Jan, a busy real estate broker, rarely takes time out for meals. She grabs a bag of chips or a sandwich for lunch while rushing to appointments. With client phone calls and paperwork stretching into the evening, dinner is generally just before bed. Jan complains of a chronically dry mouth and throat and a persistent dry cough that prompts a desire for frequent sips of water for relief. The slender, active thirty-eight-year-old feels particularly warm in the late afternoons and often wakes up hot and perspiring in the early morning. She also complains of bloating, constipation, and dry stool. Jan has signs of stomach yin deficiency.

Eating too fast or when feeling rushed, insufficient chewing, and eating too much or too soon before sleep create a burden for the stomach and spleen, producing an inefficient fuel that can leave the stomach dry, leading to indigestion, fatigue, and weakness.

Too Many Spices, Fried Foods, Coffee, and Alcohol

Dan is a busy newspaper editor saddled with a plethora of daily deadlines. He complains of an insatiable appetite and a burning sensation in his stomach between meals. He suspects an ulcer. His gums often bleed when he's brushing his teeth, and he frequently develops canker sores. His wife complains he has bad breath. Dan has classic signs of stomach fire. Although the stress of his high-pressure job fuels his symptoms, Dan's diet exacerbates the problem.

Dan eats lots of spicy food, including Indian curries, hot peppered Thai food, and Mexican dishes covered in hot salsa. He washes his well-spiced food down with several beers or martinis. French fries, commercially fried chips, and fried chicken wings are snack staples for Dan. A diet of excess fried and spicy foods, especially when combined with stress, can lead to imbalance in the form of stomach fire. Other potential stomach irritants include poor quality oils of the kind used in many restaurants, red meat, coffee, and citrus fruits.

Dieting, Starving, and Lack of Protein

The right amount and type of foods strengthen spleen Qi. Getting adequate protein foods, including poultry, meat, fish, eggs, and legumes, is particularly important. Dieting, starvation, or a low-protein diet can weaken the spleen.

When vegetarians aren't careful in selecting foods for their particular constitution, they can easily develop weak spleen Qi, with signs such as weakness and fatigue. When food intake or protein is restricted too much, the body perceives a famine and slows down its calorie-burning activities, or metabolism, weakening spleen Qi's ability to transform food into energy. If excess weight is lost and then regained, it becomes increasingly difficult to lose the weight again. Once a diet ends or when unlimited food becomes available, cravings and a tendency to overeat reflects the weakness in the spleen. When digestion is not functioning properly, energy, in the form of Qi, is not effectively extracted from food. Although calories are coming in, the body doesn't receive adequate nourishment. Fatigue and lethargy result, and we often reach for another cookie or other sweets, starches, or stimulants in an ill-fated attempt to revive our energy.

Restricted diets are virtually impossible to adhere to, and we eventually give in to temptation for forbidden breads, pastries, and cookies. By that point, it's unlikely that just one cookie will take care of a craving, and overeating or binge eating begins, which further weakens spleen Qi.

Not only does dieting weaken spleen Qi and lead to weight gain by stimulating excess appetite and cravings, it slows metabolism and thus the ability to burn off excess calories. I often hear complaints from clients that their metabolisms are too slow—they eat very little, yet they can't seem to lose weight. (Incidentally, the opposite problem—the inability to gain weight despite a calorie-rich diet—is also a sign of spleen Qi deficiency.)

Too Much Stress, Anxiety, and Antacids

One of the more common ways we weaken our spleen Qi is through worry and anxiety, which, as we know from Western studies, affects the body's digestive system. Western-trained doctors know anxiety exacerbates digestive problems, including irritable bowel syndrome and ulcers. A highly stressful situation, such as financial difficulties or a loved one's sudden

health crisis, can lead to diarrhea or constipation in someone who is otherwise healthy. TCM practitioners recognize these effects as well.

When stressed from too much work, impending deadlines, relationship
difficulties, or any other emotional or mental cause, the body reacts just as it
would if it were faced with an immediate physical threat, such as a vicious,
charging dog. Breathing speeds up, blood sugar increases, and blood and
energy are diverted from the digestive tract and into the arms and legs,
preparing the body to run like crazy or prepare to fight. From a Western perspective, anxiety causes the production of cortisol, adrenaline, and other hormones that slow digestion by diverting blood to skeletal muscles for quick
mobilization. As most of us know, this physical reaction is called the *fight or
flight response*. Mental stress readies the body for physical action, at the
expense of digestion.

Antacids are often prescribed during times of stress for relief of acid
reflux or ulcers. It has long been assumed these signs of discomfort indicate
too much hydrochloric acid (HCL) is being produced in the stomach.
Surprisingly, this condition may in fact be caused by just the reverse. HCL
is released to enable protein-digesting enzymes to better break down protein
foods. Low HCL production, however, can leave food in the digestive tract
undigested and more likely to contribute to acid reflux. In addition, we need
HCL to kill harmful bacteria that can live in the stomach. Stomach ulcers
have now been linked with an overgrowth of a harmful bacteria called heli-
cobacter pylori (H. pylori), according to Western studies. The healthy production of HCL in the stomach not only enables us to digest our food but
also prevents H. pylori from proliferating. HCL, in a sense, cooks harmful
bacteria. Instead of stimulating an overproduction of acid, stress, in many
cases, may be reducing our HCL production. Antacids, which are designed
to restrict HCL production, may thus ultimately perpetuate indigestion and
ulcers instead of healing them.[27]

Stressful situations also stimulate appetite through the release of galanin,
a chemical that stimulates cravings for fat, and neuropeptide Y, a brain
chemical that gets appetite revved up for sweets, according to Judith
Wurtman, PhD, researcher at the Massachusetts Institute of Technology.
Dr. Wurtman also says people crave chocolate because something in the
chocolate, as well as the sugar, stimulates serotonin, a brain chemical that
helps restore calm.

HABITS THAT PROMOTE GOOD DIGESTION

Just as certain habits lead to poor digestion, many others encourage strong digestion. The best way to prevent a spleen or stomach imbalance is to eat three regular meals each day, take time out for relaxation, enjoy meals in a calm state, and choose foods appropriate for your constitution, as discussed in the next several chapters. Most meals should be warm, provide a balance of types of foods, and leave you feeling comfortable and satisfied but not full.

Adequate Protein and Warming Foods

The first step to balancing someone with signs of a weak, damp spleen and poor digestion is to replace an excess of cold foods such as salads, yogurts, juices, and smoothies with warmer, cooked foods such as soups, stir fries, grilled fish or chicken, and cooked vegetables. Iced water should be replaced with room-temperature water or, better yet, hot water or hot tea.

Strong spleen Qi demands adequate (but not high) levels of protein. Individuals with certain constitutional types require some meat, poultry, or fish for balanced spleen function. For other types, a daily vegetable protein source, such as beans, lentils, or peas, is adequate. Although each us require different quantities and types of protein, most of us fare best with small amounts of poultry, fish, eggs, or meat almost every day, supplemented with daily servings of beans, lentils, peas, or soy.

Appropriate Pungent and Bitter Foods

Whether you view them as promoting digestion, resolving abdominal bloating, reducing damp sticky cholesterol deposits, or stimulating stuck Qi, pungent and bitter foods and spices get things moving. They can be either warming or cooling, thus benefiting signs of damp-cold or damp-heat when used appropriately. Bitter and pungent flavored foods can help offset the damp-forming potential of dairy products and excess meats, stimulating the movement of Qi and blood throughout the body.

Pungent foods are often warming and thus help to resolve cold, damp signs that can result from a regular diet of juices, fruits, and frozen desserts.

Warming pungent foods and seasonings include onions, garlic, scallions, rosemary, ginger, pepper, hot peppers, cayenne, dill, horseradish, wasabe, celery seeds, cumin seeds, mustard seeds, caraway seeds, fennel seeds, and coriander seeds. Cooling pungent foods are best when there are signs of dampness and heat and include broccoli, peppermint, marjoram, white pepper, daikon root, and radishes.

Bitter seasonings and foods are particularly helpful in resolving signs of dampness, including bloating and water retention, swellings, parasites and yeast overgrowth, cysts, masses, growths, and obesity. Bitter foods can act as diuretics and mild laxatives. They tend to be cooling and so can be particularly helpful when there are signs of heat. Bitter foods and seasonings include lettuce (particularly romaine), rye, radish leaves, asparagus, celery, vinegar, arugula, broccoli, broccoli rapini, chicory, watercress, kale, turnips, marjoram, oregano, and teas of dandelion leaf and uva ursi (an herb with diuretic properties from the leaf of a type of manzanita). Although not so beneficial in the long run, since it depletes our Qi and thus our energy, coffee is very bitter and, like other bitter substances, reduces dampness, acting as a diuretic and mild laxative. It is often craved for its instant but short-lived stimulation of Qi and its effect on certain signs of dampness.

Exercise

Exercise is important to stimulating the movement of Qi and critical to treating dampness, especially with excess weight. According to Chinese thought, the oxygen you breathe into the cells of your body on a brisk walk, a bicycle ride, or a hike helps to dry dampness. This theory, of course, fits perfectly with the Western admonition to do aerobic exercise regularly to burn fat and calories and to tone muscles. Incorporating movement into your daily routine is imperative to drying dampness and losing weight. Take the stairs, walk across the parking lot from your car to the store door, enjoy regular walking or hiking in the outdoors.

People in China don't do workouts exactly. They don't go to gyms. Most of them have never heard of a target heart rate or seen a Stairmaster™. Their secret is regular movement. They ride their bicycles or walk to most places. The parks in China are filled to capacity with locals practicing T'ai chi, Qi gong, and various other martial art forms. I recommend to most my clients that they incorporate thirty to forty-five minutes of aerobic exercise into their day, in the form of brisk walking, bicycling, hiking, or dancing. Adding stretching, yoga, or a martial art is even better.

Relaxation

For optimum health and digestion, it's important to incorporate strategies for relaxation into your life on a daily basis. Exercise along with designated periods for relaxation is perhaps the most effective approach. Meditation, stretching, yoga, T'ai chi, listening to soothing music, and walking in nature are a few suggestions for relaxation. I find it most helpful to choose something simple that can be practiced daily. Meditation, for instance, requires no special equipment or training. A yoga class is often a pleasant diversion from a stress-filled lifestyle. If you live near the ocean or a peaceful wooded area, a daily walk can be very calming. In addition, relaxation before, during, and following eating is essential. It allows for proper blood flow into the digestive tract, normal digestive secretions, and proper peristaltic movement to push food through the intestines. I suggest my clients take a few moments before eating to relax, clear their minds, and experience a sense of gratitude. Create a serene place for eating. Remove bills and clutter from sight. Save heated topics of discussion for later.

The Right Climate for Your Condition

Rainy, foggy, humid climates and buildings that are moldy or built into damp earth contribute to dampness and can weaken spleen Qi. If your constitution is one that tends toward dampness, you will find balance easier to achieve living in a warm, dry climate.

25. Beinfield, Harriet, and Efram Korngold, *Between Heaven and Earth*. New York: Ballantine, 1991.
26. Robert C. Atkins, MD., *Dr. Atkins' New Diet Revolution*. New York: Avon Health (1992): 4–46; H. Leighton Steward, Morrison C. Bethea, et al., *Sugar Busters*. New York: Ballantine, 1995.
27. Murray, Michael, and Joseph Pizzorno, *Encyclopedia of Natural Medicine*. New York: Prima (1998): 136.

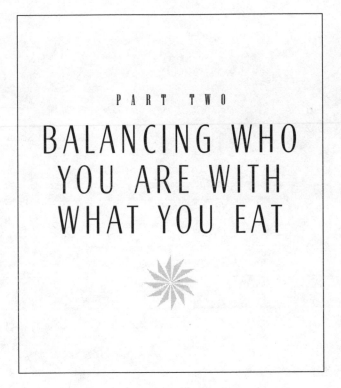

PART TWO

BALANCING WHO YOU ARE WITH WHAT YOU EAT

4

VITAL SIGNS:
IDENTIFYING PATTERNS
OF IMBALANCE

Each of us has a tendency toward a yin or yang state. Your particular mixture of yin and yang is not necessarily a reflection of illness or disease; you may be perfectly happy with your state. Being relatively yin or yang is simply a way of viewing your relationship with your environment and those around you. Usually we have a genetic predisposition toward yin or yang; however, lifestyle and environmental factors can exaggerate these tendencies or unbalance someone relatively balanced to begin with.

When challenged through stress, poor diet, too much or not enough exercise, heat, cold, or other influences, we create imbalance in our yin/yang nature. The red-faced man at the bar angrily hollering for a beer is showing signs of "excess yang." The pale, anemic woman clutching a mug of hot coffee for warmth despite sitting in a warm kitchen may have "excess yin." A person with an excess of yang will become even more yang driving in rush-hour traffic with a broken air conditioner on a blistering August afternoon. Even a person who is fairly balanced between yin and yang will likely become more yang—if only temporarily—if faced with the same anger-producing, uncomfortably hot situation.

Most of us have aspects of both yin and yang. Lisa, a client of mine, is a short, small-boned woman with soft flabby rolls of fat around her abdomen and fleshy thighs and a round, plump face. She abhors exercise and spends much of her day sitting. In these respects, she is yin. But Lisa is also a hard-driving businesswoman. She is an assertive deal-maker with the ability to raise her voice and make demands if need be. These are the yang aspects of Lisa. She exhibits both yin and yang qualities, and it's hard to tell which ones are predominant. But when we compare her to others—for instance, a large-boned, red-faced, active, hard-driving businesswoman—we can say Lisa has relatively yin attributes.

When there are signs of both yin and yang in the body, it is best to stay away from extremes, including sweets, heavily salted foods, lots of meat, spicy food, and too much alcohol. The worst foods for Lisa are foods that are damp (yin) and hot (yang). Because her body is damp, she loses weight easiest by eliminating damp, yin foods such as milk, yogurt, ice cream, juices, cookies, breads, and pasta. Her personality traits are best balanced by avoiding the hot, yang extremes: alcohol, onion rings, French fries, chips, cheese, and hamburgers. The best foods for Lisa are cooked, mildly seasoned vegetables, soups, stir-fried dishes, grilled fish and poultry, rice, corn, and small amounts of seasonal fruits.

ENVIRONMENTAL INFLUENCES ON BALANCE

Beyond yin and yang, your constitution can be further divided to reflect one or more climates, or environmental influences: cold, heat, dryness, dampness, and wind. Each of these climates further corresponds to an element, as discussed in chapter two. Cold corresponds to water, heat to fire, dryness to metal, dampness to earth, and wind to wood. For the purpose of learning about body patterns, we will focus on the environmental influences of cold, heat, dryness, dampness, and wind.

When it takes hold in the body, an environmental influence can lead to trouble. An excess of heat from one's predisposition, stress, environment, or diet, for instance, can lead to feeling too hot and irritable, as well as to high blood pressure and headaches. In this case, the environmental influence—heat—becomes what the Chinese call a "pathogenic factor." Essentially, this means that there is too much of one type of environmental influence in the body, causing a *pattern of imbalance*, also called a *pattern of disharmony.*

TCM recognizes a pattern of imbalance as a related group of signs and symptoms corresponding to one of the five environmental influences. A person who generally feels cold, has a pale complexion, and is shy and often depressed has a "cold" pattern. Someone who is always hot and has a temper and a red face probably has a "heat" pattern. If you have dry skin and hair, a dry cough, a dry throat and mouth, and hard, dry stool, it's likely you have a "dry" pattern. If you are plagued by excess weight, fluid retention, sinus congestion, or abdominal bloating, you have a "damp" pattern. Abrupt, jerky movements and shifting emotions characterize a "wind" pattern. Just as wind can occur in winter and rain can dampen a summer day, patterns can be combined in the body. Someone with a pattern of heat or cold may also develop wind or dampness. Things become more complex when such combinations of patterns exist; examples include *wind-cold* and *damp-heat* patterns.

This chapter introduces the basic patterns of imbalance and provides a diagnostic test to help you determine your constitutional tendencies; taking the test will also give you an overview of how various seemingly unconnected symptoms and conditions are linked to a common cause, such as excess cold or dampness. Once you have a sense of the pattern or patterns that may be affecting you, turn to the individual pattern chapters, which offer more in-depth discussions of the patterns and specific suggestions for balancing each one.

A Cold Pattern

The most obvious signs of a cold pattern are feeling cold despite the ambient temperature, craving warmth, and having a pale complexion as well as a quiet, withdrawn nature. Depression, apathy, and fatigue are also signs of cold. Someone with a cold pattern loves to curl up under a warm blanket in the quiet of a soft couch, perhaps with a hot chocolate.

Waking up with a full-blown head cold, complete with aches, pains, stuffy head, and runny nose, is another example of a cold pattern. When cold is combined with dampness, the result is fluid retention and clear sinus mucous. This combination is often also associated with excess body fat and a slow metabolism.

Living in a cold climate, undereating in general or eating too little protein in particular, old age, a long chronic illness, and a copious intake of ice-cold drinks, juices, fruits, frozen desserts, or other cooling foods all lead to the gradual onset of a cold pattern.

A Heat Pattern

A heat pattern is easy to spot. Signs include feeling too warm even when the temperature is not hot. If you have a heat pattern, you feel physically uncomfortable in hot weather and crave a cold drink and cool shade or an air-conditioned room. Someone with excess heat tends to have a red face and a loud voice. He or she may be irritable and prone to outbursts of temper. He or she also has a voracious appetite, with cravings often for greasy or cold foods. This person may have high blood pressure and a tendency to get headaches. Heat is also associated with fever blisters, canker sores, and red acne or rashes. The extreme side of heat is fire, although *fire* and *heat* can be used interchangeably. Fire is essentially a more serious version of a heat pattern and generally is associated with a hot climate.

Heat can be coupled with other pathogenic factors, including dampness and wind. A heat pattern of imbalance can result from a number of influences: overwork and stress, living in a hot climate, smoking, consuming an excess of alcohol and spicy, greasy, or other heating foods.

A Dry Pattern

A dry pattern can be an extension of heat. Dryness may occur when a heat pattern has gone unchecked, drying the moist, yin tissues and fluids of the body. It may also occur when the moist, yin element of the body becomes depleted—for instance, with age, at menopause, with a deficiency in essential fat, with certain medications, or with excessive worry and stress. Signs of dryness include dry lips, tongue, mouth, and throat, often with a dry cough, and the resulting desire to sip on fluids throughout the day. Someone with a dry pattern often has flushed red cheeks. He or she frequently craves sugar and may be diabetic or hypoglycemic (diagnosed as having low blood sugar). It is commonly associated with dry skin, brittle hair and nails, and a tendency toward constipation or very dry stool. Other symptoms include anxiety, irritability, and a feeling of restlessness.

Dryness is a common pattern of imbalance in perimenopausal women. An overly thin body type may reflect dryness. Yet when dryness occurs with midlife hormonal changes, including slowing metabolism and sugar cravings, it can also be accompanied by excess weight gain, particularly in the abdomen. Too much pressure and mental stress or excessive exercise can cause signs of a dry pattern. In addition, eating late at night, working while eating, making poor food choices (including following a diet too low in fat), or living in a dry climate can lead to dryness.

A Damp Pattern

A damp pattern is characterized by an aversion to wet, foggy, or humid weather conditions. Someone with a damp pattern typically retains fluid in the legs, ankles, or abdomen and experiences a feeling of heaviness as if being dragged down. Dampness may be accompanied by mental fog or muddled thinking and may settle into the sinuses, causing a sinus infection or hay fever. Dampness in the lungs may be recognized as a respiratory tract or bronchial infection. In the digestive system, dampness often includes bloating and sometimes manifests as irritable bowel syndrome or colitis.

Dampness may be found with heat or with cold. When heat and dampness co-exist, symptoms may include an aversion to hot, humid days, irritability, lethargy, bloating and gas, red inflammations, and coughing up dark yellow or green mucus. When dampness is combined with cold, signs often include an aversion to cold, a slow metabolism, a runny nose, and chills. Living in a rainy, foggy, or humid climate can lead to dampness or make a tendency toward dampness worse. Sitting on damp ground or living in a damp, moldy house can also aggravate damp signs.

A Wind Pattern

A wind pattern is often associated with serious conditions or illnesses, which sometimes have a sudden onset, such as strokes, seizures, and paralysis (Bell's palsy). The flu and colds are also wind conditions. Wind in the body, like that in nature, moves and changes. It may appear as a pain that changes locations, a sudden headache, or a rash on the chest or throat that moves to the leg or waist. Tremors, twitching, and dizziness are all signs of wind. Wind can give the other environmental influences of cold, heat, or dampness easier access to the body.

The common cold is an example of wind accompanied by either heat (fever) or cold (chills). Someone with wind-cold has a strong aversion to wind and cold and will want to stay in the warmth of the indoors. Arthritis pain in various joints that gets worse in cold weather is an example of wind-cold. When wind is combined with heat, there is the usual aversion to heat, as well as an increase in thirst, agitation, and irritability. Wind-heat can also produce dizziness, headaches, rashes, or strokes.

Too much stress, high blood pressure, and cholesterol-clogged arteries may, over a long period of time, stir up wind. A windy day or sitting in a draft may also precipitate sudden wind symptoms.

Who Are You?

Once you understand the nature of these patterns of imbalance, you can better understand why Western medicine's one-size-fits-all approach to diet or drugs doesn't work for everyone. An overweight person with a damp pattern will have trouble losing weight on a low-calorie diet if that diet includes too many damp foods. Someone with a cold pattern needs a different remedy than someone with a heat pattern, even if they have the same Western diagnosis. A headache might be from heat, cold, dampness, or wind, and the "cure" needs to be properly directed to whatever pattern of imbalance is causing the pain.

Knowing your body pattern will help you better understand who you are and what steps you need to take to achieve optimal health and weight. The ability to recognize your patterns of imbalance is a powerful tool that can help you take charge of your health and prevent disease and other problems. Your five senses and awareness of minor discomfort in your body can alert you to impending illness long before some of the most sophisticated diagnostic equipment can.

The following self-assessment tests will help you determine whether you are relatively yin or yang. They will also show you if you have signs of heat, dryness, cold, dampness, or wind. It is likely that you will have combinations of more than one pattern.

Do You Have a Pattern of Heat (Yang Pattern)?

Answer "yes" or "no" to the questions below.

1. Do you generally feel warm?
2. Are you particularly uncomfortable on hot days and generally prefer to wear cool clothing and cool weather?
3. Does your entire face and neck easily become red after exercising?
4. Are you generally thirsty, with frequent cravings for large, cold drinks?
5. Is your urine deep yellow or dark in color?
6. Do you have high blood pressure?
7. Do you suffer tension headaches?
8. Do you often get nosebleeds or bleeding gums?
9. Do you suffer from canker sores or fever blisters?
10. Do you often have bad breath?
11. Is your sleep often restless, with disturbing dreams?
12. Do you have bowel movements less than once a day?
13. Do you tend to get irritable or easily angered?

Do You Have a Pattern of Cold (Yin Pattern)?

Answer "yes" or "no" to the questions below.
1. Do you generally feel chilly?
2. Are you particularly uncomfortable on cold days and generally prefer to wear warm clothing and be in a warm room?
3. Does your complexion tend to be pale?
4. Do you generally prefer hot foods (soups, stews, hot sandwiches) and drinks rather than cold (salads, yogurt, fruit)?
5. Do you find it difficult to drink cool beverages and have very little true thirst?
6. Do you tend to feel depressed or sad?
7. Are you generally considered shy and introverted?
8. Is your urine pale or clear?
9. Are your stools generally loose?
10. Do you generally sleep curled up?
11. Do you have a slow metabolism (difficulty losing excess weight)?
12. Are your muscles soft and fleshy as opposed to toned and hard?
13. Are you frequently tired and apathetic?

Determine whether you tend toward a hot/yang or a cold/yin body pattern by totaling your score for each set of questions (one point for every "yes" answer).

If you answered "yes" to the first three questions in either category, you have a strong tendency toward that pattern. The highest scoring category indicates your body pattern tendency. If you scored almost the same in both categories (within three points), you are probably close to balance and would do best on an eating plan where warming and cooling foods are represented in a balanced fashion. If you answered "yes" to more than five questions in either category, it would be a good idea to limit extreme foods of that category. For instance, if you answered "yes" to seven questions in the heat/yang category, you will probably feel best by limiting your intake of extremely heating foods, such as alcohol, fried foods, beef, and lamb, and moderating your use of garlic, onions, and other heating foods. On the other hand, if you answered positively to seven or more questions in the cold/yin category, you will feel better by reducing frozen or iced foods, dairy products, juices, smoothies, salads, and raw vegetables.

Do You Have a Pattern of Dampness?

Answer "yes" or "no" to the questions below.
1. Do you strongly dislike damp or humid days?
2. Do you easily retain water or fluids?
3. Are you overweight and do you find it difficult to lose weight?
4. Do you often have a puffy face or creases beneath your eyes?
5. Do you feel heavy, especially in your lower body?
6. Do you frequently suffer from abdominal bloating or a feeling of fullness?
7. Do you often experience sinus or lung congestion with phlegm, a runny nose, or postnasal drip?
8. Is your urine cloudy?
9. Are you often mentally "foggy" or "fuzzy"?
10. Do you easily get short of breath?
11. Do you find it difficult to drink lots of water?
12. Are your muscles soft and fleshy rather than firm and toned?
13. Are you rarely hungry?

If you answered "yes" to any of the first five questions, you have signs of dampness. A "yes" answer to more than five questions means you have significant signs, or a pattern, of dampness. You will probably feel best by limiting your intake of highly damp foods, including dairy products, greasy foods, and sugar, as well as reducing wheat products (breads, pasta, and so on). Dampness can be combined with heat (damp-heat) or cold (damp-cold), depending on your score in the heat/yang and cold/yin categories, above. Dampness may occur in one part of the body and not in others. Abdominal bloating and indigestion suggests dampness in the digestive system but it may not be present in the limbs or other parts of the body. A head cold with congested sinuses indicates dampness in the sinuses. Obesity is dampness throughout the body.

Do You Have a Pattern of Dryness (Yin Deficiency)?

Answer "yes" or "no" to the questions below.
1. Is your skin dry?
2. Is your hair dry and scalp flaky, or do you have dandruff?
3. Do your stools tend to be dry? Do you have a bowel movement less than once a day?
4. Do you have a dry cough or dry eyes?
5. Are your cheeks frequently rosy or red in the afternoon or after exercise?
6. Do you often wake in the night feeling overly warm, sometimes perspiring?
7. Do you have a thin body type?
8. Do you frequently crave sweets?
9. Do you prefer warm or room temperature liquids rather than ice cold?
10. Do you often find yourself sipping on liquids throughout the day?
11. Are you easily irritated or frustrated?
12. Are you restless or anxious?
13. Do you have a poor memory?

If you answered "yes' to any of the first five question, you have signs of dryness. Common causes of this pattern are stress, overwork, and too much time in dry, centrally heated (or air-conditioned) buildings. You will probably feel best by increasing moistening foods such as therapeutic oils (see chapter eleven), soy products, black beans, soups, stews, yams, oily fish, and pumpkin seeds. Limit your intake of spicy foods.

Do You Have a Wind Pattern?

Answer "yes" or "no" to the questions below.
1. Do you have an aversion to cold weather or wind?
2. Do you frequently develop head colds with shivering, sneezing, coughing, and runny nose?
3. Are you prone to the flu?
4. Do you ever develop paralysis in any part of your body?
5. Do you experience convulsions or seizures?
6. Do you have itchy areas on your skin?
7. Do you have an itchy sensation in your throat?
8. Do you sometimes experience dizziness or vertigo?
9. Have you had a stroke?
10. Do you feel nervous?
11. Are you easily irritated?
12. Do you have pains or rashes that move around?
13. Do you experience any signs of dryness? (See the dry pattern test, above.)

If you answered "yes" to more than three question, you have signs of wind. Wind is often an acute condition that can appear suddenly, such as a cold, or worse, sudden vertigo, a stroke, or Bell's palsy. Although often combined with imbalances of heat, cold or dampness, wind is more serious than the other environmental influences. Wind conditions often result from long-term imbalances that weaken the immune system, deplete our yin fluids, clog and harden the arteries, and/or stress and overheat the liver.

BALANCING PATTERNS OF DISHARMONY

For the most part, nutrition and lifestyle hold the key to achieving optimum health and balance. But first you need to know whether you have patterns of cold, heat, dryness, dampness, or wind. Once your pattern or patterns are determined, you can choose the foods, herbs, and cooking techniques that, along with appropriate lifestyle changes, will help restore balance—preventing more serious health problems and, in many cases, healing illness.

The Chinese principles for balance and healing are straightforward: When a pattern of heat exists in the body, the best remedy is to provide cooling foods and lifestyle changes. When a pattern of cold exists in the body, warming remedies are needed. Restoring moisture relieves a pattern of dryness, and, conversely, drying remedies are called for in treating a pattern of dampness.

Using the Balancing Nature of Foods

Food offers a powerful way of supplying warming, cooling, moistening, or drying properties to the body. The effects of foods go beyond their physical temperature or moisture content. Although the temperature of a food can impart cooling or heating effects, foods can also be energetically cooling or heating, which means the nature of that food (be it eaten cold or warm) carries its characteristic property deep into the body. Damp and dry qualities of foods, likewise, have little to do with their moisture content; rather, their moistening or drying properties have more to do with stimulating or inhibiting secretions.

Iced water, frozen yogurt, and chilled fruit juices are cooling, yet so is cooked spinach, tofu, crab, and eggplant. Served warm or cool, these foods impart a cooling quality to the body's tissues. Garlic, cinnamon, lamb, and alcohol are hot; even when served cool, they drive warmth into the stomach and blood. A cold beer or freezer-cold vodka, despite its temperature, is heating to the body. Tofu, spinach, whole wheat, and black beans are moistening to a dry pattern. Turnips, many green vegetables such as broccoli, and whole rye are drying foods, particularly helpful for damp conditions. Most bread, even in the form of toast, is relatively damp, not dry as you might expect.

Fruits and vegetables tend to be more cooling than meats, so a diet based on lightly cooked vegetables, salads, and fruits is going to be more beneficial to someone with a pattern of heat than would a diet rich in meat. Raw foods are generally more cooling and damp than the same foods cooked. Thus raw foods may benefit someone with a heat pattern but be a problem for someone with a damp-cold pattern.

You can also use the energetic properties of foods to shift your yin/yang state of mind or mood. For instance, choosing the right foods at lunch can facilitate a productive, energized afternoon. Stimulating, yang foods, such as fish, poultry, beef, or eggs, promote the release of catecholamines, brain chemicals that leave us alert, energized, and productive. Too much damp-producing food, such as bread, pasta, or potatoes, on the other hand, can leave you tired and mentally foggy through the afternoon.

When called upon to deliver a convincing presentation or to argue your side of a case, you may choose to bring out stronger, yang, heating energy by eating beef for lunch. When I first began giving nutrition presentations, I was often nervous and even felt a little spacey beforehand. Using Chinese principles, I started eating a salted, hardboiled egg, a heating yang food, just before going in front of my audience. This method helped tremendously in grounding and focusing my energy and allowed me to feel stronger (more yang) and self-assured.

On the other hand, the right dinner can help take the edge off a stressful day. Since vegetables and whole grains balance a yang pattern, common after a stressful day of work, incorporating these foods into an evening meal would enable you to feel mellower and less anxious for the evening. This type of meal stimulates serotonin, the brain chemical that has been shown to boost feelings of happiness, calm, and focus. Or, if you're having a dinner party, you can serve your guests foods to either lighten their spirits or stimulate serious debates. Champagne, fruit, and salad lift spirits, whereas salty dishes, meats, and cheese are likely to promote more thought-provoking conversation.[28]

Adjusting Your Lifestyle to Create Balance

Just as your food choices can control your health and mood, so can your lifestyle choices. The most important lifestyle practice for health is balance: balance between work and play, activity and sleep, exercise and rest, mental effort and a calm or still mind.

Developing a routine that includes a regular sleep schedule and three meals per day is a basic but powerful lifestyle practice. Ideally, 25 percent of your food should be taken at breakfast, 50 percent at lunch, and 25 percent at dinner. TCM experts consider the common practice of making dinner the largest meal of the day as one of the worst dietary practices among Americans. Overeating at night can create stomach heat and stagnation of food in the stomach, which imbalances digestion and therefore spleen health.

Engaging in the right amount of exercise for your individual needs is also critical for optimum health. Too little is likely to lead to dampness and overweight, indigestion, lethargy, and low moods. Too much activity, however—say from training for a marathon—can deplete vital yin fluids, resulting in dryness and perhaps irritability. Ideally, you should choose an appealing form of aerobic activity, such as walking, jogging, swimming, cycling, dancing, or hiking, and make it a regular, enjoyable part of your routine. Activity should be stopped or modified whenever you experience pain or discomfort.

Those with a damp pattern will benefit by including aerobic activity daily or almost every day. Dampness, like a wet towel, needs air to dry. Aerobic activity, full breathing, and a dry climate are helpful in balancing a damp condition.

The most common lifestyle situation that leads to poor health in our society is overwork and stress. The type-A, hard-working, stressed-out business executive often depletes his or her moist, cooling yin fluids by spending too much time at an office engaged in work. These habits can ultimately lead to signs of dryness and heat, including redness in the face, a dry mouth and throat, irritability, restless sleep or insomnia, and sugar cravings.

Appropriate lifestyle changes for those who have signs of dryness or heat are taking time out to relax, working fewer hours, and spending time in a cool place, perhaps near water. Lighter forms of activity, such as yoga or meditation and leisurely walks in nature, perhaps three to five days a week, are particularly helpful.

HELP YOURSELF TO BETTER HEALTH

Once you figure out your condition, learning how to use the appropriate foods for balance is fairly straightforward. In the following chapters, you will find descriptions and self-assessments to enable you to identify general patterns of imbalance in your body. I've provided balancing suggestions for each pattern, highlighting the foods and cooking methods you should use and those you should avoid. I also include tips on exercise and lifestyle for each pattern.

However, this book is not meant to take the place of a Western or Chinese doctor's expertise in diagnosing or treating disease. The tools provided here are designed to give you a general reading on your overall state of health. The self-assessment tests above, as well as those in the pattern-specific chapters, will enable you to understand the signs of cold, heat, dryness, dampness, or wind in your body. In some cases, you'll be able to determine an imbalance in your liver, stomach, or digestive system. But if you are experiencing a chronic condition of any sort, acute discomfort or pain, or a variety of different signs, such as heat in one place and cold in another, you should seek professional help. Oriental Medical Doctors (OMDs) and licensed acupuncturists (LAcs) are trained in special diagnostic techniques to clarify signs and obtain more specific information. In addition to prescribing dietary changes, these professionals employ acupuncture and medicinal herbs to specifically and powerfully target the area of imbalance.

For information about finding an OMD or LAc, see chapter twenty three.

---

28. Champagne and wine, because they come from fruit, tend to induce calm and lift our spirits in the short run, including while we are drinking them. Champagne, in particular, is uplifting because the rising bubbles stimulate and carry Qi, or energy, upwards, Overuse, however, leads to signs of heat, especially in the liver.

5

THE BIG CHILL:
TREATING A COLD PATTERN

Kathy is a thirty-five-year-old wife and mother. When she first comes to see me about losing weight, she is bundled in a sweatshirt and jacket, even though it's a sunny, warm day. Her face is pale and puffy, her hips and thighs wide and fleshy. She wants to lose at least forty-five pounds.

Kathy is shy and withdrawn. Getting her to talk about her health requires tenacity on my part. She reluctantly admits she is tired and depressed much of the time. Some of her problem stems from inactivity. "It's hard for me to motivate myself to exercise," says Kathy. "I'm so exhausted and down all the time." Fluids accumulate in Kathy's legs, leaving her feeling heavy, as if weighted down by bags of water. She often experiences lower-back pain. She feels most comfortable alone, often avoiding social activities and friends.

After asking a lot of questions, I discover Kathy catches colds every few months, more often in winter, and when she does, she suffers a persistent runny nose and sneezing. Her muscles ache and she gets nasty chills. During a recent medical check-up, Kathy was told she was anemic.

In an effort to lose the excess weight that's plagued her since high school, Kathy tries to eat salads and fruits whenever possible. She eats a fat-free cold cereal with skim milk and orange juice for breakfast. Kathy rarely eats meat, yet she often gives in to the temptation for hot, creamy, and cheesy pasta dishes, buttered noodles, warm bread with butter, and pizza. She also loves salty foods and often succumbs to her urge for hot, salty French fries. She also craves hot coffee drinks and hot chocolate.

Kathy's difficulty losing body fat, retention of fluids, fatigue, depression, and feeling cold are signs of a cold pattern of imbalance; that is, she has too much yin (moisture and cold) relative to yang (heat). When water puts out fire, or yin suppresses yang, a pattern of cold emerges. Cold may or may not reflect an actual disease in Western medicine, although if left untreated, it is likely to become a recognized illness.

Kathy's diet exacerbates her cold pattern by placing a heavy emphasis on cooling foods while leaving out sufficient warming foods. The way to balance for Kathy is to eat more warming, or yang, foods and to engage in physical activity to buoy her spirits, stimulate metabolism, and increase the formation of muscle, a yang tissue.

I suggested to Kathy that she replace salads with sautéed and stir-fried vegetables. I urged her to eat more hot soups and stews and to replace pasta dishes with grilled chicken, beef, lamb, and fish, plus cooked vegetables. For breakfast, I had Kathy switch from her usual cereal and juice to eggs and hot tea. Hot, cooked foods and meats gave Kathy the warming, stimulating effect she wasn't getting from salads, bread, cereals, and pasta dishes.

I also recommended exercise to balance her cold pattern. Regular afternoon walks up and down the hills of her neighborhood are helping her shed the excess weight and firm and tone her legs. Exercise also helps boost her energy levels and instill a sense of self-confidence. After changing her eating and exercise patterns, Kathy actually "came out of her shell," said one of her friends. Instead of avoiding friends and social events, Kathy began to warm up to her friends and engage in more contact with others.

SIGNS OF A COLD PATTERN

Cold is a yin pattern associated with the element water and with the winter season. Many of the qualities of a cold pattern reflect those of winter. Cold qualities are contracted, rigid, moist, and quiet. If you have a cold pattern, you are frequently chilly regardless of the outside temperature, you may retain fluid or water, your sinuses may often be congested and your nose runny, and you're probably fatigued, apathetic, insecure, or depressed. You tend to be pale, soft spoken, and introverted, and you prefer to be left alone, curled up and still under a warm blanket on a soft couch, perhaps with a warm snack.

A cold pattern is characterized by inactivity, low metabolic rate, depressed mental activity, poor circulation, weakness, and malaise. In Western medicine, a person with a cold pattern may be diagnosed with low thyroid function, weak adrenals, or anemia. Cold-pattern types generally crave warm food, drinks, and weather. They order hot coffee or hot tea instead of soft drinks or iced water. They tend to move to warm, desert areas such as southern Arizona or southern California. They are the ones wearing sweaters and jackets when others are dressed in short-sleeved shirts.

If you have a cold pattern, you may have weak spleen (digestion) and experience bloating and gas. Food seems to take forever to digest. Your body's metabolism is slow, due in part to your tendency to be sedentary. Exercise warms the body by stimulating circulation and muscle formation. Muscle generates more heat than fat, so building muscle will warm the cold pattern and burn fat. Diminished metabolism and less muscle may make it difficult to burn excess fat.

Cold blocks the circulation of Qi, the yang life force that warms and stimulates the body. When Qi isn't moving adequately, fatigue and malaise set it. People with cold and damp patterns often crave warm food, as well as chocolate, coffee, or alcohol—generally bitter or pungent substances containing caffeine or other chemicals that stimulate Qi and thus both body and mind, providing a temporary feeling of renewed energy.

Cold constricts tissues, including blood vessels, causing poor circulation. Thus, if you have a cold pattern, you may have cold hands and feet. Cold is also rigid, like ice. Someone with a cold pattern may feel stiff with painful joints. According to TCM, "Retention of cold causes pain." Rheumatoid arthritis, especially in old age, is often a sign of cold reaching into the joints. A cold pattern most commonly elicits arthritis pain in the hands, arms, feet, knees, lower back, and shoulders. For women, pain in the reproductive organs can lead to debilitating menstrual cramping. When cold affects the stomach, stomach pain and sometimes vomiting result. In the intestines, cold causes diarrhea.

Other signs of cold include clear watery discharge from the nose, clear urine, and clear vaginal discharge. Asthma, when characterized by watery or foamy mucous in the lungs, is a cold pattern. (In contrast, the dark yellow or green mucous produced from a deep cough is a sign of heat.)

The common cold, when it includes shivering, sneezing, runny nose, coughing, and body aches, in Chinese medicine is a cold pattern. It is said to be combined with the pathogenic factor *wind* (described in chapter nine) to produce *wind-cold*.

In TCM, the corresponding emotion for the element water is fear. Someone with a pattern of cold may appear to have greater insecurities than other types. He or she may be fearful about losing his or her job, insecure about losing a spouse, or excessively worried about harm coming to his or her children. I was once introduced to a man named Rob. One of the first things I noticed was his bright, pale complexion and a look of panic on his face. My first thought was that he was terribly afraid of something or startled. Upon getting to know him better, I learned he suffered from chronic lower-back pain and weak knees, both signs of a kidney imbalance. His nature was introverted, and he tended to be depressed. I later learned he was terrified of losing his wife, so he went to great lengths to investigate her contacts and daily routine, eventually driving her to seek a separation.

THE KIDNEYS' ROLE IN A COLD PATTERN

Cold is associated with the element water. The associated organ systems, appropriately enough, are the kidneys and the bladder, organs that regulate water balance in the body. According to Western physiology, the primary function of the kidneys is to regulate body fluids by forming urine. They filter out and eliminate body waste from fluids. In TCM, the kidneys and the bladder are functions, not just organs—the kidney function includes the actual kidneys and the adrenal glands, but its significance is much more profound. The kidneys are often referred to as the "Root of Life." They are the foundation of the yin (fluids) and yang (heat) for all other organs of the body. Kidney yin moistens and nourishes all the tissues of the body. Kidney yin fluids include hormones, intracellular fluid, skin oils, saliva, vaginal fluid, semen, and digestive secretions. Kidney yang provides warmth and energy and a balance to yin for all other organs. All other organ systems rely on the kidneys.

In TCM, kidney health is synonymous with qualities of youthfulness: youthful energy, acute vision and hearing, fertility and sexual appetite, healthy offspring, strong bones and teeth, thick vibrant hair. Because of their role in hormone and semen production, the kidneys support all reproduction, including the reproductive organs, sperm, ovum, libido, and all reproductive activity. The lubricating nature of kidney yin prevents inflammation, including that of joints. Arthritis can result from a deficiency of kidney yin and is often aggravated by cold. Although cold and dampness are both yin, each is influenced independently; we may become deficient in one with signs of excess in the other. This is particularly the case in old age, when our moist, yin fluids begin to dry up at the same time our youthful yang flame begins to wane, leaving us yin deficient and cold. This pattern that accompanies aging is known as kidney-yin deficiency or kidney weakness.

When kidney yin is depleted through stress, poor diet, or old age, we begin to dry up, producing fewer hormones, fewer skin oils, and less moisture for elimination. Our skin becomes dry and wrinkled; our hair becomes dry; our estrogen, testosterone, and progesterone levels drop; digestion slows; and our ability to convert food to energy declines. A cold pattern or kidney weakness also affects hearing. Interestingly, TCM says the stress of noise weakens the yin aspect of the kidneys, which leads to hearing loss. As we age and our kidneys grow weaker, our ability to hear declines. From a Western standpoint, noise, over time, just blunts our ability to hear. We take it for granted that hearing diminishes with old age.

ARE YOU SUSCEPTIBLE TO A COLD PATTERN?

While anyone can develop a kidney imbalance and a disordered water metabolism, those most susceptible are the water-element archetypes. Physically, the water-element archetype tends toward big bones and a large head. The hips, pelvis, and legs are sturdy and sometimes fleshy. Women water archetypes who become out of balance tend to take on a pear shape and complain of a slow metabolism.

At her best, the water type exhibits a vivid imagination and is curious, bright, and introspective. A philosopher by nature, this type shines light on difficult subjects and discerns meaning in life events. The water type is independent.

When out of balance, the water type becomes withdrawn, insecure, and negative. Her body may appear stiff and inflexible, as if hardened by cold. He or she may become cynical, sarcastic, and detached, pulling away from friends and family. Metabolism tends to be slow, so weight gain is easier than with other body types. Fluid retention often swells the ankles, legs, and other areas of the body, driving up blood pressure. The joints often become stiff and sore.

COLD PATTERN				
Element	**Season**	**Organs**	**Emotion**	**Sense Organ**
Water	Winter	Kidney, Bladder	Fear	Ears/Hearing

SIGNS OF A COLD PATTERN

Lists are in alphabetical order unless otherwise noted.

Key Characteristics
Note: Listed in order of significance.

aversion to cold weather and craving warmth

pale complexion

craving warm foods and often spicy flavors

lack of thirst

clear urine

sleeping in a curled-up position

Secondary Characteristics

clear sinus or vaginal discharge

difficulty sweating

fatigue, lethargy

flabby muscles

loose bowel movements

pain in lower back or knees

rigid body, stiffness

sharp pains, sensitive to pressure

slow metabolism

tendency to be depressed

tendency to be fearful

tendency to be insecure, passive

lack of desire to exercise

reluctance to talk

weak appetite

withdrawn, yielding

Potential Diseases

anemia

arthritis, especially in hips and knees

asthma

emphysema

head colds

tumors, nodules, lumps

CAUSES OF A COLD PATTERN

As previously suggested, some people are by their very natures and physiques prone to cold patterns. However, anyone may at any time develop such a pattern. A cold pattern is more likely to arise when one is living in a bitterly cold climate, spends too much time in an air-conditioned building, or is exposed to a draft, but the pattern may also reflect eating too many cold foods or too few warming foods as well as a lack of exercise. Though fears and insecurities are frequently *symptoms* of a cold pattern, an exaggerated fearfulness or isolation may actually contribute to cold signs.

Cold is the natural progression as we age. As children we are most active, vital, and spirited (yang). As youth mellows into old age, we become less active, cooler, more yin as the yang flame of our youth diminishes. Older people are often seen wrapped in extra sweaters because they get cold easily. We also get stiffer with age—our joints become less mobile and sometimes arthritic. Thus, while a balance between warming and cooling foods is important throughout life, it becomes increasingly so as we age.

Drinking iced water with meals, sipping on smoothies and shakes, and frequently eating ice cream puts out the fire of digestion, contributing to a cold pattern. Too many energetically cold foods, including salads, raw fruits, and juices, can also be overly cooling for digestion and the body. Certain foods, including raw vegetables and most raw fruits, although they may not necessarily be cold to the touch, impart a cooling quality to the tissues of the body. Feasting on raw salads, cucumber slices, carrots, and celery sticks can lead to bloating, loose stools, gas, fatigue, and other symptoms of a cold pattern in anyone.

During my early twenties I was convinced a meatless diet of salads and raw fruits was the way to eternal health. I ate huge bowls of raw lettuce, spinach, sliced cucumbers, tomatoes, carrots, and sprouts, only to be left desperately wanting sweets. My favorite dinner was a baked potato with nonfat yogurt and a huge salad. Between meals I feasted on peaches, melons, bananas, oranges, and grapes, all the while craving cookies and muffins. Occasionally I went on a juice or watermelon fast. In time my abdomen became bloated and distended. I felt gassy and uncomfortable. I was tired, depressed, and chilled, and, despite my low calorie diet, my weight was climbing. According to Western doctors, nothing was wrong. "I suggest you exercise more and eat less," advised one endocrinologist I went to about my escalating weight.

Eventually I went to a Chinese doctor, who told me I needed more meat and fewer raw foods. I resisted his advice, having read for years that a raw-foods vegetarian diet was the healthiest way to go. One day, out of desperation, I tried chicken. It almost immediately buoyed my energy and lifted my spirits. After integrating chicken as well as other meats into my diet, sugary foods lost their magnetic appeal. I was finally able to lose the excess body fat and tone up.

In addition to raw and cold foods, a cold pattern and kidney weakness can be exacerbated by eating too many salty and bitter foods. Salt, in some instances, is very cooling. Packaged and processed foods, such as soups and frozen meals, tend to be especially loaded with salt. Soy sauce and other condiments are also salty and should be used in moderation. Cooling bitter foods, including lettuce, alfalfa sprouts, cucumber, and arugula, also tend to be cooling and are best minimized in someone with cold signs.

FOODS TO FIGHT WINTER COLD

Anyone can feel cold during winter, regardless of our patterns. In colder months, we tend to draw our energies inward for introspection, reflection, and quiet. We stay indoors more, feel less inclined to activity, cook more meals at home, and crave warmer, cooked foods, including, for most people, chicken, beef, and lamb, the most warming of foods. Hearty chicken, lamb, and beef soups and stews seasoned with onions, leeks, and garlic not only taste best in winter but are also especially nourishing for the kidneys and for warming us when it's cold outside.

It's no coincidence that during winter we spice our desserts with the warming flavors of cinnamon, nutmeg, and cloves. We like hot teas and soups instead of lemonade and iced water. Most cold-season vegetables are warming, including root vegetables, parsnips, and rutabagas, as well as sweet, orange, fleshy winter squash, especially when baked and sprinkled with cinnamon. We have a natural tendency to choose warming foods to fight off excess cold.

REMEDIES FOR A COLD PATTERN

Stoking the body's yang energies is the way to balance for someone with a cold pattern. That may mean exercise, asserting oneself, and eating warming foods while reducing cooling foods. Sometimes you need only do one of these things to notice a change; sometimes you need to do all three.

Aerobic exercise, including walking, jogging, bicycling, hiking, rowing, climbing, or dancing, is beneficial because it stimulates Qi, gets blood circulating, and generates warmth. In someone with a pattern of cold, the stimulation of blood flow is desperately needed to the limbs and extremities. In addition, activity stimulates lymph and mobilizes fluids, helping to reduce swellings common in a cold pattern. Movement boosts metabolism, helping to burn excess fat. It also raises endorphins, the brain chemicals that elevate mood, providing relief from depression and low self-esteem, both of which are common with a cold pattern. Strength training, including weight lifting or use of resistance machines, adds muscle, a yang tissue and thus warmth, to the body.

Foods beneficial for balancing a cold pattern include beef, chicken, lamb, salmon, eggs, and warming herbs. Warming grains include oats, sweet rice, quinoa, and basmati rice. Oatmeal with cinnamon and walnuts makes an ideal breakfast for someone with a weak kidney function and a cold pattern. Basmati rice is a delicious, fragrant, nutty grain and the perfect complement to the warming nature of a curried dish or a beef or chicken stir fry with ginger and garlic. Sprouted grain breads are particularly helpful in moving sluggish Qi. Sprouted grains are whole, uncooked grains allowed to soak in liquid until they germinate, or sprout. According to TCM, this process changes their digestive properties, rendering them less damp.

Although most vegetables aren't considered particularly warming, many are nonetheless helpful in stimulating Qi and thus energy as well as in reducing excess weight and fluids in someone with a damp-cold pattern. Vegetables provide nutrients such as B vitamins, potassium, and magnesium that help regulate fluids in tissues and elevate energy and mood. From a Chinese perspective, almost all vegetables provide properties that move the congested Qi often associated with a cold pattern. Excellent choices include cabbage, kale, mustard and turnip greens, ginger, garlic, onions, scallions, chives, and cayenne, all of which are warming as well as stimulating to sluggish Qi, thereby enhancing energy and circulation. Other warming vegetables include parsnips and most other root vegetables, broccoli rabe, and winter squash. Cooking renders vegetables less cold and more easily digested and absorbed than raw vegetables. The higher temperatures of sautéing, grilling, baking, broiling, and stir frying, in particular, make vegetables less cooling.

Adding the warming qualities of spices such as garlic, ginger, onions, scallions, turmeric, or black pepper in the cooking process is particularly healing for a cold pattern. Ginger, a very warming seasoning, works as an anti-inflammatory for cold-type arthritis. (Ginger is recognized by natural Western medicine as a remedy for arthritis pain, as well as for stomach pain and vomiting.) Capsaicin, a naturally warming constituent of cayenne, is another common arthritis remedy. This substance is often found in topical creams formulated to reduce joint or muscle pain. Adding pine nuts, toasted sesame seeds, toasted sesame-seed oil, mustard seeds, cumin, and turmeric are also flavorful ways to impart warmth to vegetable dishes.

Although most raw fruits should be minimized for those with a pattern of cold, moderate amounts of cooked fruits—such as peaches cooked into oatmeal, apple sauce cooked with cinnamon, or a warm berry cobbler—are acceptable ways of including fruit in the diet.

Some raw fruits can be enjoyed, especially during warmer months or during periods of moderate exercise. A few fruits, including peaches, cherries, dates, and plums, are actually warming (yet also damp). Pears, melons, bananas, and persimmons, on the other hand, are especially cooling and should be avoided by those with a cold pattern.

Warming sweeteners can be used in moderation by those with a cold body pattern. Acceptable options include barley malt, molasses, and rice syrup. Stevia is a non-caloric sweet herb beneficial to all patterns. However, stay away from refined white and brown sugars. Although they're heating, they are also overly damp and contribute to excess body fat, which, as we know, tends to be a problem for the cold body type. Both types of sugar are also associated with depression and low energy, conditions to which cold body types are especially prone.

The following lists of foods are those *particularly* helpful to someone with a cold pattern; *they are not comprehensive lists of acceptable foods*. A balanced diet for this pattern includes a broad range of neutral and even slightly cooling choices used appropriately. Many cooling foods, such as spinach or tofu, can be made less so by being sautéed with garlic, ginger, or other warming spices. Only those foods listed under "Foods and Beverages to Minimize" should be eliminated or used only occasionally.

BALANCING REMEDIES FOR A COLD PATTERN

Vegetables

asparagus	parsley
broccoli rabe	parsnips
cabbage	red cabbage
kale	rutabagas
mustard greens	turnip greens
onion family (onions, chives,	
garlic, leeks, scallions)	winter squash

Grains

basmati rice (white or brown)	quinoa
buckwheat	spelt
kamut	sprouted grain breads
oats, oatmeal	glutinous rice

Protein Foods

Note: Listed from most to least warming

lamb	red-fleshed fish
venison	salmon
beef and other red meats	shrimp
chicken	turkey
pheasant	trout
eel	black beans
anchovies	fava beans

Nuts, Seeds, and Cooking Oils

Note: All are okay for a cold pattern but the following are especially warming. Always use fresh. Oils should be cold or expeller-pressed and organic.

almonds	pine nuts
coconut	sesame seeds/oil, (toasted or untoasted)
flaxseeds	sunflower seeds/sunflower oil (choose the high oleic
	variety because it holds up to cooking better.)
hemp seeds	walnuts/walnut oil (unheated)
olive oil	

Foods for Strengthening Kidney Function

black beans	goat-milk yogurt and cheese
black sesame seeds	kidney beans
broken bone soup (see chapter twenty two)	pork (lean)
chicken	sesame oil
flaxseeds	walnuts
fish	

Cooking Methods

bake	sauté
broil	stir fry
grill	use warming spices

Beneficial Activities and Situations

exercising aerobically	strength training
socializing with others	warm weather, sunshine

Foods and Beverages to Minimize

Note: Some cooling foods are okay for a cold pattern with the addition of something warming, for example, spinach cooked with garlic.

crab	milk
cucumbers	raw fruits and juices
eggplant	peppermint
ice cream, frozen yogurt, or other frozen desserts	salads
iced water and other iced beverages	tofu (especially uncooked)
kelp and most sea vegetables	yogurt
melon	

Situations to Avoid

air-conditioned buildings	drafts
cold bodies of water	isolation
cold climates	

6

HOT AND BOTHERED:
TREATING A HEAT PATTERN

Jack, a solid, burly, fifty-six-year-old newspaper editor, asked me for nutrition advice to help lower his elevated blood pressure and cholesterol levels. His doctor informed him he was headed for a heart attack. Upon further questioning, I learned Jack also suffers from tension headaches. He often wakes in the night, restlessly tossing and turning, dreaming of deadlines and work-related problems. The ruddy-faced, gruff-voiced editor works ten to fifteen hours a day, demands near perfection from his staff, and yells fiercely, often losing his temper, when things don't go as planned. He's generally too warm, never dressing in more than a short-sleeved cotton shirt and often reaching for sodas to quench his nearly constant thirst. Jack's favorite meals are steaks and hamburgers, especially with French fries chased with a Pepsi. After work, Jack heads to his favorite bar where he drinks several beers.

Jack has a heat pattern of imbalance, sometimes called *excess* or *full heat*. Relaxation, in addition to increasing water intake and cooling foods while decreasing warming foods, helps a pattern of excess heat. After a scare with heart pain, Jack began cutting back on his hours at work. He started taking three-day weekends to drive to nearby mountains to read and play golf. Jack replaced steak dinners with more fish, cooked vegetables, and salads, and slowed down on the alcohol and saturated fats. He added fruit to his diet and cut out the French fries. Within a few months, Jack had lost twenty pounds, reduced his blood pressure to normal, and acquired a more relaxed demeanor.

SIGNS OF A HEAT PATTERN

A heat pattern is associated with the fire element and with the summer season. When a pattern of disharmony with heat signs emerges, many of its characteristics reflect the nature of heat. Consequently, a heat imbalance is more likely to appear during the summer months. Someone with signs of heat tends to feel uncomfortably warm and dislikes hot climates. He dresses in cool clothes and often will become irritable on a hot day or in a hot room. His face is generally red—the color associated with the fire element—and he may perspire easily. He craves cool weather; hot summers bring out the worst in him, causing mental and physical restlessness.

According to TCM theory, the effects of excess heat are seen most often in the heart, vascular system, and mind. Heat rises, so signs of a heat imbalance are often in the upper body. The rising nature of heat in general can lead to signs such as splitting headaches, bloodshot eyes, ringing in the ears, a bloody nose, gum disease, mouth sores, dizziness, high blood pressure, and increased risk of heat attack. A person with excess heat may experience a bitter taste in the mouth as well as bad breath. Appropriately, the cooling nature of mint, often used in breath mints, is the ingredient of choice for neutralizing bad breath.

A heat pattern may also characterize infection with a fever. Excess heat in the body can cause bleeding, including bleeding gums, or hemorrhage, including certain cases of hemorrhoids. When excess heat exists in the body, the blood lost from a sore or injury is bright red. Some types of arthritis involve a heat pattern; when hot weather or a meat-rich diet aggravates arthritis, heat is generally the culprit.

Summer heat is a particular type of heat that results from overexposure to external heat from a hot summer day or too much time in a sauna or hot tub.

Signs of summer heat are high fever with heavy sweating, a headache, and heat exhaustion. It may also include shortness of breath and production of phlegm. In extreme cases, it can result in dehydration and delirium.

Heat can affect specific areas of the body. When heat associated with the heart becomes too strong, it affects the lungs, causing dryness. The result is often a dry, hacking cough, thirst, and sores in the mouth and nose. Any red eruption in the body, including hives, canker sores, fever blisters, herpes, eczema, and acne, can be signs of heat in the body. Red inflammations, swellings, and rashes are signs of excess heat. Dark yellow urine is also a sign of heat somewhere in the body.

Heat can be particularly problematic when it affects the liver. When the liver becomes hot, it can't function properly. Because of its influence over the spleen and digestion, liver heat can lead to burning gastric ulcers, indigestion, and colitis. When the liver's role in clearing hormones from the body is impaired, anger and emotional highs and lows, including PMS, often result.

In women, liver heat can manifest as irritability and other PMS symptoms, as well as early, heavy menstruation with bright red blood. If left unchecked, such profuse bleeding, a yang condition, may result in anemia and eventually its opposite: a cold, or yin, pattern. The painful, burning urination associated with a bladder infection is also a sign of heat.

A heat pattern is also characterized by a voracious appetite and thirst. Someone with a heat pattern doesn't like to miss meals. If heat builds up in your stomach—as from excess alcohol and spicy foods or too much stress—you may experience a chronic burning sensation in the stomach, which registers as hunger. My clients with stomach heat often tell me they have an out-of-control appetite, which leads to overeating. Someone with a heat pattern can eat large portions at mealtime and often will crave cold food and drinks, such as ice cream, sodas, and cold beer. It's easy for someone with heat excess to gulp a large glass of cold soda, water, or beer.

People with heat patterns often have cravings for the stimulating effects of alcohol. However, while a cold beer or icy cocktail appeases excess heat in the short run, it ultimately makes a heat condition worse. Similarly, eating ice cream often feels soothing, temporarily relaxing the stomach and relieving feelings of tension and agitation; unfortunately, the fat and sugar (both heating) of ice cream further contribute to a heat pattern, while the cold temperature makes the stomach heat up because it has to work harder to offset the cold. To make matters worse, the cold nature of ice cream also interferes with optimum digestion, or spleen function, leading to bloating and other symptoms of indigestion.

The corresponding emotion for the element fire is translated as joy, which doesn't quite convey the meaning intended in TCM. More accurate is the idea of the overexcitement that comes with too much partying or always being stimulated. Constant excitement or a state of excessive stimulation can weaken the heart and the fire-type individual, precipitating signs of heat: headaches, migraines, or even heart attacks.

Someone with a heat imbalance is easily irritated and quick to anger. His temper may be short, and when he gets overly agitated, his sleep becomes restless with disturbing dreams and his words may make little sense. He may also feel frustrated or stuck in life. The sound associated with fire is laughter. Inappropriate or frequent laughing, or the inability to laugh, are signs of an imbalance in the fire element. The corresponding sense organ is speech or the tongue. Speech problems, including stuttering or incoherent speech and an inability to tell the truth, also indicate imbalances in the fire element. People with excess heat are often anxious and extremely sensitive, with swings from happiness and laughter to sadness and crying. Allowed to continue over a long period of time, a heat pattern begins to erode mental and physical health. The risk of stroke, heart attack, and mania increases in someone with a heat pattern.

THE HEART'S ROLES IN A HEAT PATTERN

Heat is associated with the element of fire. The principle organ correlated with heat and fire is the heart (yin). The heart's yang partner is the small intestine. The Chinese say that the fire element "rules" the heart and the small intestine. When an excess of heat exists, the heart is said to be out of balance. Someone who has a fire imbalance is likely to have weakness in his or her heart, perhaps suffering from angina, atherosclerosis, or other forms of heart disease. An excess of heat leaves one at greater risk of stroke. He or she may also have digestive problems, including diverticulitis or constipation.

In TCM, the heart is also the mental, or emotional, center, said to "house the spirit." When heat depletes the body's soothing, moistening yin aspect, our spirits can become restless and on edge. Characteristic signs of excess heat, then, include agitation, irritability, and delirium (or mania)—signs of a disharmonious spirit. Someone with an excess heat pattern tends to be very restless and agitated. He may lose his temper and shout easily. His sleep is often restless, with disturbing dreams.

ARE YOU SUSCEPTIBLE TO A HEAT PATTERN?

Virtually anyone can develop a heat pattern of disharmony. The individual most prone to heat, however, is the fire element archetype. At his best, this individual is affectionate, warm, friendly, open, and charismatic. He's the life of the party, impassioned by excitement. He loves a good time. He is also able to be intimate and show empathy toward others. He is intuitive and sensitive. Physically, he is soft and willowy, with graceful hands and feet. His legs and arms tend to be long. When unbalanced from overeating in general or too many spicy foods in particular, excess alcohol, or too much excitement, his face gets red.

When the fire element individual gets out of balance, he most easily develops the signs and symptoms of excess heat in the body: He becomes hot easily and may perspire heavily. He may be restless and irritable, have disturbing dreams, or develop fever blisters. His speech becomes impaired in some way, perhaps with stuttering or nonsensical statements. He may become very talkative and laugh at the end of every sentence or be unable to laugh at all.

HEAT PATTERN				
Element	**Season**	**Organs**	**Emotion**	**Sense Organ**
Fire	Summer	Heart, Small Intestines	Joy/Excitement	Tongue/Taste

SIGNS OF A HEAT PATTERN

Lists are in alphabetical order unless otherwise noted.

Key Characteristics
Note: Listed in order of significance.

aversion to hot weather and craves coolness   dark yellow or red urine thirst or desire for cold beverages

red complexion

easily irritated or angered

restless and agitated

Secondary Characteristics

bad breath

bitter taste in mouth

bloodshot eyes

bloody nose

dream-disturbed, restless sleep

fast pulse

frequent canker sores or fever blisters

hypersensitivity

inappropriate laughter or crying

talkative/loud voice/shouting frequently

tendency to be aggressive

tension headaches

voracious appetite

Potential Diseases

arthritis

bleeding gums, gum disease

colitis

eczema

migraines

hemorrhoids

high blood pressure

mania

gastric ulcers

heart disease

CAUSES OF A HEAT PATTERN

Stress is well known in Western science to increase risk of heart disease and, in TCM, to give rise to all the signs of a heat imbalance. Anger and frustration, in particular, are causes as well as symptoms of heat. Western science recognizes that overwork, toxic relationships, and money worries—those situations that spark anger, frustration, and stress—can raise damaging levels of stress hormones such as adrenaline and cortisol, driving up blood pressure and cholesterol levels and stimulating an excessive appetite. These emotions can also precipitate headaches, sleepless nights, skin flare-ups, and irritability—all symptoms of excess heat.

In TCM, stress, anger, frustration, overwork—as well as poor diet, alcohol, and drugs—are recognized as contributing to heat. If these contributors are allowed to continue, the energy of the body—its Qi—become stuck or stagnant. When static, this life force, in turn gives rise to liver heat, which leads to even more anger, rage, and frustration—as well as a number of physical health conditions, such as heart attack and stroke.

Too much excitement can also fuel heat signs. Too many parties, too much sex, excessive drinking and eating, and using recreational drugs tax the heart and can contribute to excess heat. Alcohol and tobacco are particularly heating.

Overeating in general and especially eating too much at night creates heat and burdens the heart. Foods, in particular, that can exacerbate a heat imbalance include refined white and brown sugar; coffee; fried, greasy, or oily food; too much red meat, chicken, cheese, or eggs. Spices, including black pepper, hot chilies, ginger, cinnamon, garlic, and onions turn up heat in the stomach, further increasing appetite, perpetuating the cycle of overeating, and increasing heat signs.

A high-meat diet is unbalancing for someone with a heat imbalance for several reasons. Not only is meat itself a heating food, but also its high-protein and phosphorus content interfere with calcium absorption and utilization. Meats are also low in magnesium. Calcium and magnesium are calming minerals; they play a role in lowering elevated blood pressure. Magnesium is essential for production of serotonin, a brain chemical associated with good moods. Coffee consumed at meals interferes with the absorption of calcium. Refined sugar, alcohol, excess salt, and smoking also cause calcium to be excreted in the urine.

FOODS TO FIGHT SUMMER HEAT

The summer season and hot climates tend to bring out heat signs in everyone, regardless of pattern. Increasing cooling foods, such as salads and fruits, and decreasing warming foods, such as meats, fried and fatty foods, is beneficial for everyone at such times. Salads, raw vegetables and fruits, steamed vegetables and fish generally taste best in summer or when it's hot. Foods available in summer are generally the most cooling. This makes sense from an ecological perspective, as the foods most suited for consumption during a certain time are grown in that area at the appropriate time of the year. For instance, meat, which is more available than vegetables in winter, is heating, while fruits and vegetables grown during the summer are cooling. Such summertime foods include lettuce, watermelon, honeydew melon, tomatoes, cucumbers, summer squash, eggplant, and bell peppers.

Poor quality fats, including old or unsaturated oils used for frying, margarine, and other hydrogenated fats and saturated fats contribute to excess heat as well. Most margarine is hydrogenated, a process of adding hydrogen molecules to an oil to give it a stable shelf life and to make the consistency buttery. Unfortunately, the process of hydrogenation, sometimes called *partial hydrogenation* on food labels, renders vegetable oil much like a saturated fat, in that it clogs arteries and increases the risk of heart disease, but worse. According to results from a large Harvard health study, which looked at food intake and health of 80,000 nurses, hydrogenated fats, including margarine, were fourteen times more potent than saturated fats at increasing risk of heart disease. Dr. Walter Willett, epidemiological researcher at Harvard School of Public Health, estimates 30,000 premature deaths each year in this country can be attributed to eating hydrogenated fats. Other studies, too, suggest margarine may be worse for heart health than using butter or even lard.

Hydrogenated fats are now found in everything from commercial salad dressings to crackers, cookies, breads, flour tortillas and commercially baked products. Fast-food restaurants fry French fries, onion rings, chicken pieces and other foods in hydrogenated oils. These foods are particularly harmful because they have been cooked in oils that have been at a high heat for extended periods and reused. Overheating oils causes formation of harmful chemicals called free radicals, which have been implicated in cancer and heart disease. Any product that lists margarine, "hydrogenated" or "partially hydrogenated vegetable oil" on its label should be avoided. Excess saturated fats from fatty cuts of beef or lamb, poultry skin, butter, and lard can also lead to heat signs and heart problems.

REMEDIES FOR A HEAT PATTERN

The best treatment for excess heat is to take time out for mental and physical relaxation. Replace basketball or competitive cycling with swimming or golf. Lead a simpler life. If worry about work is preoccupying your mind, cut back on your workload. Take steps to make your home a restful, peaceful place. Scale back on the parties and alcohol. Read more. Take up gardening or another relaxing hobby. Maintain a program of physical activity such as walking, bicycling, or swimming to keep stress-related chemicals at bay in the body. If you smoke, stop. Eat a light evening meal to help reduce stomach heat.

Acupuncture and cooling herbs also help restore balance to someone with a heat pattern. Water is critical for those with heat signs—copious amounts of cool (but not cold) purified water should be consumed daily. Foods should be cooling in nature. In general, that means a predominance of lightly cooked or raw vegetables and fruits as well as whole grain products. Salads, raw cucumber slices, lightly cooked greens, melon, soy foods such as tofu and miso soup, yogurt, and most seafood are harmonizing for someone with a heat pattern.

Those who have subsisted on a steady diet of burgers, fries, steaks, and other rich, fried, or greasy foods often find a primarily raw-foods diet to be healing and calming. Focusing on salads, raw vegetables and fruits, or even a modified fast of fruits, vegetable juices, and salads, when used appropriately, can provide welcome relief from irritability, headaches, voracious appetite, and other signs of heat. Cholesterol and blood pressure levels will plummet when the focus is on raw vegetables and fruits with little added fat. Such raw food diets are beneficial for a short period of time to balance years of an overly heating diet. They should not, however, be thought of as long-term remedies. Remember balance. Just because you have heat in your body does not mean a regimen of *all* cooling foods is the perfect diet. Don't fall into the no-fat or all-raw food fads. Raw foods are healing programs and are beneficial as long as they leave the body feeling balanced. Large-meal-sized salads loaded with raw spinach, carrots, and tomatoes or large intakes of fruit, all-fruit meals, or juice, are very cooling to the stomach and dampening to the spleen and may, in time, lead to digestive problems and a new set of health problems: cold pattern or damp pattern. Before signs of weakness, fatigue, cravings, bloating, indigestion, or loose stool begin, balance out the raw with more cooked vegetables. A small salad with lunch and dinner, a few carrot sticks, and two pieces of seasonal fruit in a day may be a good place to start. (More raw produce may be helpful for certain individuals.)

Fluids, including drinking generous quantities of water, are important to someone with a pattern of heat. Cooking foods in broth or other liquid at low temperatures renders them more moist and cooling than frying, sautéing, searing, baking, pressure cooking, or grilling does. A generous intake of soups and food cooked in liquids is helpful in reducing excess heat. Poaching, braising, steaming, and boiling are the most beneficial cooking techniques for a heat pattern.

Very warming foods should be minimized in someone with a heat pattern. These include alcohol, coffee, fried foods, lamb, beef, and spicy foods. Other heating foods include cayenne, hot peppers, cinnamon, black pepper, chives, scallions, refined sugars, peanuts, walnuts, garlic, chives, nutmeg, cloves, rosemary, and turmeric.

The taste associated with fire, or the heart, is bitter. The bitter flavor imports a cooling quality. Cooling bitter foods, including leafy greens: romaine and other lettuces, celery, dandelion greens, arugula, broccoli, and certain herbs are said to help control heat.

Greens are also excellent sources of calcium and magnesium, both calming and cooling minerals. In fact, the addition of a calcium and magnesium nutritional supplement can further help in facilitating calm in someone overstimulated by a heart imbalance or with a pattern of heat. Magnesium, in particular, is a cooling, calming mineral, one well known in Western medicine to play a role in heart health. In fact, supplements of magnesium are used to treat angina (heart pain), high blood pressure, and congestive heart failure. Studies have found people who die from heart attacks have lower than normal heart magnesium levels, and intravenous magnesium is now a treatment for acute heart attacks. Calcium supplements help in some cases to lower elevated blood pressure. Magnesium can be helpful taken as a supplement at levels of 350 to 400 milligrams per day. Calcium can be helpful when taken in doses of 400 to 800 milligrams per day, or even higher if desired.

The following lists of foods are limited to those *particularly* helpful to someone with a pattern of heat; *they are not comprehensive lists of acceptable foods*. A balanced diet for this pattern includes a broad range of neutral and even slightly warming choices used appropriately. In fact, many of the vegetables list in chapter five, for a cold pattern, can also be used for those with heat signs since vegetables are more cooling than most other foods. Only those foods listed under "Foods and Beverages to Minimize" should be eliminated or used only occasionally.

BALANCING REMEDIES FOR A HEAT PATTERN

Those with a heat pattern should drink lots of cool (not cold) bottled or purified water.

Fruits

apples	melons (especially honeydew)
bananas	mulberries
blueberries	papaya
cranberries	pears
grapefruit*	persimmons
kiwi fruit	strawberries
lemons, limes*	tomatoes

* although cooling to the body, citrus fruits may cause stomach heat for some people

Vegetables

alfalfa sprouts	radishes
bamboo shoots	sea vegetables
bitter melon (a Chinese vegetable)	snow peas
bok choy	spinach
broccoli	squash, summer
carrots	sweet potatoes
cauliflower	swiss chard
celery	tomatoes, tomato juice
cucumbers	turnips
dandelion greens	watercress
eggplant	water chestnuts
lettuce, especially romaine	white mushrooms
Napa cabbage	white mushrooms
pumpkin	

Grains

amaranth	millet
barley, whole	rye
blue corn	whole wheat, especially the germ and bran
corn	wild rice

Protein Foods

Note: Listed from most to least cooling.

beans, especially mung, kidney, lima, and navy beans	shellfish, especially clams and crab
soy products, including edemame, tofu, tempeh, soy milk, miso soup, soy cheese, and soy yogurt	egg whites
white fleshed fish, especially butterfish, perch, sardines, herring, mackerel	yogurt (goat's milk is best)

Nuts, Seeds, and Cooking Oils

Note: Always use fresh, use sparingly. Oils should be cold or expeller-pressed and organic.

canola oil	olive oil
flaxseeds	pumpkin seeds

hemp seeds

high oleic safflower or sunflower oil

soybean oil (not for cooking)

Cooking Techniques

poach

simmer

steam

use raw

Activities

eating light evening meals

meditating

practicing yoga

reading

stretching

taking time off from work

walking near a beach, lake, or rive

Foods and Beverages to Minimize

Note: A small amount of heating foods is okay when used in a meal of primarily cooling foods, for example, tofu and spinach sautéed with garlic.

alcohol

coffee

French fries, chips, and other fried foods

greasy foods

margarine and other hydrogenated
vegetable oils

lard, butter, and other saturated fats

spicy foods and seasonings, including
black pepper, hot chilies, garlic,
chives, dried ginger

peanuts, peanut butter, walnuts, pine nuts

poultry, dark meat and skin

red meat, especially lamb

refined sugars

very hot (temperature) foods

poor quality or old oils

Activities and Situations to Avoid

anger-inducing situations

excessive stimulation or excitement

frustrating situations

overeating

smoking

working long hours

7

DESERT DAYS:
TREATING A DRY PATTERN
OR YIN DEFICIENCY

Jan, a forty-one-year-old real estate broker, is irritated because I am
five minutes late for our nutrition counseling appointment. I notice Jan's
cheeks are bright red and rough. Her skin and hair look dry. She is fidgeting
and appears anxious.

She comes to see me because she says she craves sweets and, although
she appears slender, she complains of getting "fat around the middle." Jan
particularly craves frozen yogurt, diet sodas, and fruit drinks. Despite generous lunches, Jan longs for a frozen dessert in the afternoon. She needs to eat
often or she feels agitated, hungry, and light-headed. Even though she's only
forty-one, she also complains of menopause symptoms including irritability,
forgetfulness, missed periods, and waking up in the early mornings hot and
sweating. She also tends toward constipation, especially when stressed.
Sitting across from me in my office, Jan shifts restlessly in her chair. She
readily accepts a glass of water and takes many sips but doesn't finish it.

Jan shows signs of dryness, or *yin deficiency* in Chinese vernacular. Our yin aspect is the cooling, calming, moistening element of the body—our juice or lubricant. Our yin aspect has to do with actual bodily fluids, including blood, hormones, skin, and scalp oils, eye fluid, moisture in the intestines, vaginal secretions, and saliva. According to TCM, healthy moisture, or fluid, is thought to originate in the kidneys. Thus, when our yin becomes depleted, the condition is referred to as *kidney yin deficiency*. With kidney yin deficiency, we deplete precious lubricating oils throughout the body, including in our skin and hair, as well as the fluids in our mucous membranes and our intestines.

Jan's symptoms lessened when she began to relax, take time off from work, tend to her garden, and play more with her children. A shift in her eating patterns was also essential. She replaced snacks of cookies, candy, and ice cream with whole-grain breads with soy or goat cheeses, crackers with hummus, and goat's milk yogurt. She reduced coffee and cut back on sodas and alcohol. She added more yin-nurturing foods to meals, including salmon, trout, tofu, flax seeds, and cooked spinach, and began adding olive oil in cooking. The changes left Jan more like her old self: cheerful, calm, and relaxed.

SIGNS OF A DRY PATTERN AND THE ILLUSION OF HEAT

Dryness is a pathogenic factor sometimes associated with the dry season, or autumn. It is often precipitated by external forces, such as a dry climate or dry, centrally-heated buildings. It may also arise from poor eating patterns, which tend to leave the stomach dry. Unlike a full-blown yin deficiency, which affects the entire body, dryness takes place in specific areas of the body, such as the stomach, the skin, or the hair. If left untreated, however, dryness can lead to a kidney yin deficiency, though yin deficiency isn't always preceded by dryness.

Because our yin fluids help cool the body, when they become depleted, signs of heat often occur. Excess heat, however, is not the true cause of this condition; rather, a lack of cooling yin fluids makes it feel as if there is too much heat in the body. Thus kidney yin deficiency is sometimes called "empty heat" or "the illusion of heat." Hot flashes at menopause, for instance, although suggesting heat in the body, are in fact caused by a deficiency of cooling yin fluids, not an excess of heat. This pattern of imbalance usually occurs with advancing age or when we are under stress, especially when accompanied by poor eating habits.

Jan shows signs of kidney yin deficiency. Her signs of dryness and heat occur even though she has no actual excess yang, or heat, in her body; rather, her moist, cooling, calming fluids have been depleted by modern stresses, overwork, worry, and poor food choices. Yin balances the yang in the body; with a deficiency of yin, it appears as if there is too much heat in the body because the yin (water) is no longer sufficient to balance the yang (fire). The remedy for such a pattern requires not so much cooling the yang influences as replenishing or nourishing the depleted yin fluids.

For the purposes of this chapter, we'll focus on yin deficiency dryness, since TCM addresses and treats this condition more often than a dry pattern.

SIGNS OF YIN DEFICIENCY DRYNESS

Heat and the illusion of heat share similar symptoms but there are nevertheless clear differences in signs and treatment. While someone with heat is hot most of the time, the illusion of heat is characterized by feeling particularly hot in the afternoons or waking up in the night hot and sweating. With a yin deficiency, often the palms of the hands and feet become hot and perspire. This symptom tends to alternate with cold hands and feet. Someone with an excess heat pattern has a red face, whereas someone with empty heat tends to have an ashen complexion with red cheeks. With empty heat comes a vague sense of tension and anxiety whereas someone with excess heat is much more agitated.

"I feel dried up," says Jan. As with excess heat, empty heat is characterized by a dry mouth and throat and frequent thirst; however, with an empty heat pattern the urge is for small, more frequent sips of fluid in an attempt to replenish diminished body moisture. Someone with yin deficiency often prefers room-temperature or even warm water whereas someone with true heat signs prefers large intakes of cold water. The common practice of carrying around water bottles or drinking the requisite eight to ten glasses of water a day may seem healthful, but these habits can also be a sign of dryness and depleted yin. Rather than quenching it temporarily with lots of water, the optimal remedy includes yin-nourishing foods.

When depleted or deficient, we lose the precious moistening oils that keep our skin smooth and soft and hair glossy, and we may develop dry skin and dandruff. Stools become hard and dry, often leading to constipation. Dry-eye syndrome can occur. We may have a persistent, dry cough. When the lubricating fluids in our joints dry up, rheumatoid or osteoarthritis and other types of inflammation may develop. When hormones dry up, infertility and loss of libido may result. Symptoms of menopause, including hot flashes, cessation of menstruation, arthritis, skin and vaginal dryness, and irritability, are signs of kidney yin deficiency.

A very thin person, especially in old age, is generally yin deficient; however, not everyone with yin deficiency is thin—weight gain can occur if the warming, drying influence of yang energy supplied by the kidneys also becomes deficient. A person with a dry pattern may perhaps experience a rapid weight loss without changing his or her diet or exercise patterns. In Western medicine, this is symptom of diabetes. He or she may experience frequent hunger, urination and thirst, signs of diabetes mellitus. When the yin is diminished, one develops cravings for sweets, especially cool, moist desserts, including frozen yogurt, ice cream, pudding, and fruits.

Other conditions associated with empty heat include hypertension, hypoglycemia, chronic eye problems, and nervous disorders. A generalized sense of anxiety and a feeling of being unable to relax are also common signs of empty heat. This dry pattern leaves a vague sense that something isn't quite right. There's a sort of generalized worry: Did I forget to bring something with me? Will the check arrive today? Are the kids getting enough at lunch?

THE LUNGS' ROLE IN A DRY PATTERN

The yin organ associated with dryness is the lungs. The yang partner of the lungs is the large intestine. The lungs govern vital energy, or Qi, which influences the circulation of blood through the network of blood vessels and arteries. The lungs receive Qi from breath and combine it with the Qi from food, distributing it throughout the body. The lungs are also said to distribute body fluids to the skin and hair, maintaining their moisture and the function of perspiration. If the lungs lack Qi, the pores won't hold perspiration in place, and frequent, chronic sweating can occur, even with a dry pattern. Healthy lungs are required for the integrity of the skin, including its moist, smooth texture, as well as the luster and sheen of the hair. Healthy skin, in turn, protects us against infection from bacteria and viruses. The colon, or large intestine, releases waste from the body. If it is failing to do its job, the skin and hair can also suffer. When our lungs become dry, a dry hacking cough may develop, and ultimately more serious lung disorders, such as tuberculosis, may occur.

The corresponding emotion for dryness is grief or sadness. Because of its association with the lungs, sadness can have a powerful effect on one's breathing and lung health. Chronic sadness, as from the loss of a loved one, can weaken the lungs, sometimes resulting in shallow breathing or, worse, lung diseases. I once worked with a client whose father and husband both passed away within one year. Soon afterwards, she came down with a lengthy bout of pneumonia, which recurred several times. When she felt she had adequately grieved her losses, her lung health improved. Long, unresolved grief contracts the lungs, interfering with breath and the health of the lungs, including their ability to disperse yin fluids throughout the body.

ARE YOU SUSCEPTIBLE TO A DRY PATTERN?

Dryness, as an environmental factor, corresponds to the element metal. Metal-type people tend to be organized, efficient, and disciplined. They are often calm with little outward display of emotion. Metal types don't exhibit the passion or tendency toward anger that a wood or fire type does. Their minds are analytical, methodical, and sometimes critical. Doctors and scientists tend to be metal types. They appreciate systems, structure, order, and control. This may be reflected in a neat, orderly house, immaculate car, well-organized desk, and adherence to systematic procedures. Her mind is logical and ideals are pure. When the metal type becomes unbalanced, he or she may appear overly ritualistic, strict, too disciplined, and perfectionistic. He or she may become rigid about diet and exercise routines. Physically, an unbalanced metal type tends to develop dry skin, hair, and mucous membranes, a dry cough, a stiff spine, and constipation.

DRY PATTERN				
Element	**Season**	**Organs**	**Emotion**	**Sense Organ**
Metal	Autumn	Skin, Hair	Grief, Sadness	Nose/Smell

SIGNS OF A DRY PATTERN OR KIDNEY YIN DEFICIENCY

Lists are in alphabetical order unless otherwise noted.

Key Characteristics
Note: Listed in order of significance.

feeling hot in afternoons or waking up hot at night	dry skin and hair or dandruff
red cheeks	constipation
frequent thirst for small sips of fluids	irritability
heat in palms of the hands or in feet, especially at night	

Secondary Characteristics

anxiety, worry	nervous disorders
dry cough	ringing in ears
dry eyes	sugar cravings
fidgeting	

Menopause Symptoms

anxiety	insufficient vaginal lubrication
hot flashes	night sweats

Potential Diseases/Conditions

arthritis	hypoglycemia
diabetes	infertility
hypertension	tuberculosis

CAUSES OF A YIN DEFICIENCY DRY PATTERN

While one's environment, a prolonged illness, menopause, and advancing age can contribute to a yin deficiency, a host of other factors—most of them lifestyle choices—can also lead to this type of dryness. Women seem particularly susceptible to depletion of yin, and they are most in need of balancing their yin aspect.

Work

City life, with all its demands and hurried pace, pulls us from our moist, calm center. Regular computer use, exposure to too much electromagnetic radiation, and airplane travel dries our skin and respiratory systems, obvious signs of depleting yin. Paul Pitchford in *Healing with Whole Foods* points to yin deficiency as a result of several generations in the industrial era, with all the stress, noise, competition, and heating, yin-depleting substances in our diet, such as alcohol, coffee, cigarettes, and synthetic drugs.[29]

More women are experiencing yin deficiency than ever before because we're pushing aside yin-nurturing domestic activities to type away at computer keyboards or chase paper over desks in sterile office buildings. We develop anxiety about deadlines. We're working too many hours, then taking home our worries to fill our hours off.

We have little time left for cooking meals. We head out for drinks and dry bar snacks in the evenings instead of standing in the fragrant steam of a simmering soup. We grab a piece of toast or cup of coffee as we head for the car in the morning instead of relaxing over the sweet mix of hot oatmeal with cinnamon. We travel in the drying compartments of planes. We swallow yin-depleting medications for pain, anxiety, and depression. Somehow, women need to find balance between work and activities that nurture our yin.

Likewise for men, working too many hours or too much worry, spending excessive amounts of time in front of a computer screen or in a dry, centrally heated building, and other stresses of the city can deplete their yin.

Stress

Stress is one of the major associations with kidney yin deficiency. From the Western viewpoint, stress exhausts the adrenal glands, the corresponding organ to the Chinese kidneys. We know stress causes excessive production of adrenaline and noradrenaline, hormones produced by the adrenal glands that lead to increased blood pressure, heart rate, and metabolism, plus sugar cravings—all signs of heat. This reaction to stress was originally designed to mobilize the body for short term emergencies—either a fight or the ability for quick flight. Adrenal hormones provide a burst of energy by elevating blood sugar, boosting the heart rate, and increasing blood flow to the muscles. The intended burst of activity, while thwarting a physical threat, returns hormone levels to normal. Unfortunately, what happens to many of us in modern society is we are chronically stimulating this fight-or-flight response and doing little in the way of physical activity to dissipate its effects. Instead of our adrenal hormones being released to help us escape a wild boar, they are released when we're at a report deadline or finding ourselves in traffic late for a meeting. Over time, our adrenals become weakened from overuse, and we become fatigued.

In addition to adrenaline, the chemical cortisol is released from our over-stimulated adrenal glands. Both chemicals cause sugar cravings in an attempt to boost flagging energy level. Cortisol stimulates production of a chemical called neuropeptide Y (NPY), a nerve chemical that stimulates cravings for carbohydrate-rich foods, especially sweets. Cortisol also causes the release of insulin, a hormone that controls blood sugar levels. Sugary foods only worsen the effects of stress by further stimulating the energy-draining, kidney-depleting hormones.

From a Chinese perspective, when our yin is diminished, we often experience cravings for sweets, especially cool, moist deserts, including frozen yogurt, ice cream, pudding, and fruits. Candy, cookies, and other sources of refined sugar can be temporarily satisfying because of their damp nature. Women often crave the cooling, bitter quality of chocolate, especially during PMS, when yin fluids are further depleted. Unfortunately, the damp, heating property of sugar often ends up causing *damp-heat* in the digestive system, leading to abdominal bloating and weight gain. The heating property of sugar and the bitter, cooling quality of chocolate further exacerbate signs of heat and dryness. Excess sugar weakens the kidneys, the organ system that regulates water in the body, and our source of yin fluids. The Chinese kidneys correspond with the Western adrenal glands, which are perched on top of the kidneys and produce secretions that enable the kidneys to function. Sugar overstimulates the adrenal glands, causing high amounts of adrenaline to be released—and the pattern continues.

Sports and Recreation

Over-exercise can also deplete yin. Running marathons, partaking in triathlons, and hiking too long and too far depletes moisture and yin. One of my clients, a woman approaching menopause, found that when she engaged in the rigorous training required to compete in marathons, she developed hot flashes. When she cut back on running and ate more yin-replete foods, her hot flashes stopped. Vigorous exercise on a hot day is especially depleting. Walking on sidewalks and asphalt, instead of playing in grassy fields and lush parks, also diminish our yin, whereas the earth and plants restore yin.

Smoking marijuana and tobacco and taking prescribed, over-the-counter, and recreational drugs also tend to deplete our precious fluids.

Sex and Reproduction

Too much sex can be a significant cause of yin deficiency. How much is too much? It varies from person to person. According to Giovanni Maciocia in *The Foundations of Chinese Medicine*,[30] sexual frequency should decrease with age, but in general twice a day is acceptable in our twenties, once a day in our thirties, once every three days in our forties, once every five days in our fifties, and once every ten days after sixty. The kidneys are the source of all essences and the organ system associated with reproduction. Along with loss of semen is loss of yin. In women, abortions also drain yin. The more abortions, the more yin is lost. Bearing children depletes some yin, although not as much as abortions do. Having too many children or too many abortions for one's constitution can lead to yin deficiency.

Menopause

As women age, the role of the kidneys in supplying the body with moist yin fluids, including estrogen and progesterone, declines. Symptoms of menopause, including hot flashes, cessation of menstruation, arthritis, skin and vaginal dryness, and irritability, are signs of kidney yin deficiency. Weight gain can occur when the warming, drying (metabolism-boosting) influence of yang energy supplied by the kidneys also becomes deficient. Declining thyroid hormone levels at midlife are ofen the Western explanation for slow metabolism and weight gain. Digestive secretions also lessen with diminished kidney yin, and abdominal bloating may occur. Diminishing blood (yin) causes skipped periods or blood flow that is more scant and brownish in color.

Coffee

Like many extreme foods, including sugar, hot peppers, and alcohol, coffee is a paradox. It is warming and energizing at first, but ultimately it cools and dries the body, leaving us cold and tired, signs that the kidneys are weakened. The bitter-and-pungent flavor compounds in coffee give us the temporary warmth and burst of energy that so many of us enjoy. The caffeine rush of a cup or two of java, from a Chinese perspective, is the feeling of Qi rapidly moving upward and out of the body. The diuretic action of coffee burdens the kidneys, stimulating the loss of warming Qi and fluids, which, over time, contributes to dryness and kidney yin deficiency. Indeed, the fatigue and dark circles under the eyes of heavy coffee drinkers are signs that the kidneys are overstimulated. Additionally, the cooling properties of coffee tend to weaken not just the kidneys but the spleen, thereby weakening digestion as well.

REMEDIES FOR A DRY PATTERN

The most helpful way to restore the moist, cooling qualities of yin and relieve the experience of dryness and anxiety is to relax and work less. Enjoying time in peaceful places, especially at the ocean, a lake, a stream, or an area of lush vegetation, feels calming because it restores yin. Getting back to nature moistens us. Spend time in your garden or walk in a nearby park. Dig your hands into moist soil to plant tender green seedlings. Moreover, deliberate long, slow breathing can calm emotions and thoughts, as well as improve some of the problems caused by dryness. For those suffering dryness due to external dry forces, such as climate or living conditions, reducing the amount of time in these environments (for example, working fewer hours in a dry office building) would be helpful.

Dietary recommendations for restoring yin are similar to those for treating a heat pattern but with an emphasis on the addition of essential oils. As with a heat pattern, a generous intake of bottled or purified water is important. With yin deficiency, a more frequent intake of water is best. Heating foods, including fried and greasy foods, poor-quality fats, spicy food, and alcohol, should be avoided. Bitter foods, including bitter greens, chocolate, and rye, should be used sparingly. Energetically cooling foods, especially cooked vegetables and tofu, as well as fish are important additions. The diet should be supplemented with flaxseeds, flaxseed oil, hemp seeds and oil, or fish oils. Raw vegetables and fruits, although helpful for those with signs of heat, may be a problem for those with empty heat. The kidneys are said to loathe cold. Thus, if you have a yin deficiency, eating too many raw foods can increase digestive problems.

Balancing sugars and proteins is generally called for with deficiency of yin. Refined sugars, including candy, sweet breakfast cereals, baked foods, ice cream, and frozen yogurt should be reduced. If you eat sugary foods daily, try limiting yourself to a sweet treat every other day.

Reaching for cookies and candy is often a sign more protein is needed. Sugar and protein are one of the most basic yin/yang food pairs. They balance each other. Protein from such sources as fish, poultry, eggs, and beans nourish the kidneys, providing moisture for the body. Protein foods also stimulate the brain chemicals necessary for energy, thereby decreasing cravings for sugar. Some neurochemists speculate that cravings for sugar, coffee, and chocolate may be an attempt to stimulate the brain chemicals, including catecholamines, such as dopamine and norepinephrine, lacking from a diet too low in protein. Protein foods also stimulate the adrenal glands and adrenaline production, providing energy and elevating mood. A balance of protein is critical, however. Just as with too much sugar, too much protein will overtax the adrenals and the kidneys.

Particularly good foods for replenishing a deficient yin pattern are black or kidney beans, fish, chicken, chicken soup, pork, cooked vegetables, whole grains, sea vegetables and essential fats—particularly omega-3 fats. Chicken and pork and additional essential fats are helpful foods to heal the illusion of heat but may aggravate a true "excess heat" pattern.

Fatty fish, including salmon, mackerel, trout, herring, and sardines, with their rich omega-3 fat content, are particularly helpful in restoring yin fluids. Other beneficial sources of omega-3s include flaxseeds, flaxseed oil, hemp seeds, hemp oil, pumpkin seeds, walnuts, oatmeal, and supplements of fish oil.

Beneficial grains include millet and barley. The bright yellow, tiny, round grains of millet make a delicious hot breakfast cereal. Millet also makes a savory alternative to rice. Barley is perfect in soups, as a breakfast cereal, or as a replacement for pasta or rice.

Black or kidney beans cooked with sea vegetables such as kombu, wakame, or sea palm and prepared with oil are excellent for restoring yin fluids. Beans made into soup with sesame or olive oil and served with sautéed vegetables are an ideal yin-rebalancing meal. Black sesame seeds, toasted in a pan and sprinkled on vegetables, soups, chicken, or eggs, also make for a beneficial yin tonic. Tofu, miso soup, soy milk, soy cheeses and soy yogurt, and tempeh (a fermented soy yogurt product prepared and used much like tofu) are beneficial, as are goat milk products—especially yogurt.

Good vegetables for a yin imbalance include spinach, eggplant, sweet potatoes, green beans, and beets. Try soy or goat cheese melted on sautéed spinach and mushrooms. Or add roast sweet potatoes, beets, and white potatoes with olive oil in a hot oven..

Just as it is with excess heat, magnesium is a beneficial mineral for the illusion of heat. It helps stabilize blood-sugar levels and thus, from a Western standpoint, helps hypoglycemia or diabetic symptoms. Western symptoms of magnesium deficiency—anxiety, headache, sugar cravings, insomnia, constipation—are similar to empty heat symptoms in Chinese medicine. Magnesium helps restore calm by reducing an anxiety peptide, a protein molecule in the brain. Good food sources of magnesium are whole grains (especially wheat germ), almonds, walnuts, and green leafy vegetables. Magnesium can be helpful taken as a nutritional supplement at levels of 350 to 400 milligrams per day. Chromium, another essential mineral for stabilizing blood sugar levels, is helpful when there are sugar cravings and blood-sugar fluctuations characteristic of hypoglycemia or diabetes. A supplement of 300 to 500 micrograms is useful.

Bitter foods, including lettuce, rye, dandelion greens, celery, turnips, and chamomile tea, are cooling and beneficial to a heat pattern; however, they tend to be too drying for someone with the illusion of heat.

The following lists of foods are limited to those *particularly* helpful to someone with a dry pattern or yin deficiency; *they are not comprehensive lists of acceptable foods.* A balanced diet for this pattern includes a broad range of neutral and even slightly drying choices used appropriately. A few foods for dry signs are also listed under remedies for a damp pattern because they are balancing to both. In other words, some foods can both help reduce excess moisture and supply moisture when needed. Only those foods listed under "Foods and Beverages to Minimize" should be eliminated or used only occasionally.

BALANCING REMEDIES FOR A DRY PATTERN OR YIN DEFICIENCY

Those with yin deficiency should drink lots of cool (not cold) bottled or purified water.

Fruits

apples	mandarin oranges
avocados	mulberries
bananas	pears
blackberries	plums
cantaloupe	pineapples (for a thin body type)
figs	pomegranates
grapes	raspberries
kumquats	

Vegetables

carrots	sea palm
cucumbers	sea vegetables (seaweed)
bean sprouts	spinach
beets	sweet potatoes
eggplant	Swiss chard
green beans	tomatoes
Kombu	wakame
Napa cabbage	water chestnuts
parsnips	winter squash
potatoes	yams

Grains

Note: It is especially important that grains be well cooked and well chewed.

amaranth	quinoa
barley, whole	rice, sweet
kamut	spelt
millet	whole wheat (except for those with abdominal bloating or digestive trouble)

Protein Foods

Note: listed from most to least moistening.

black beans and kidney beans (when prepared with oil and sea vegetables)	pork (for a thin body type)

fish (especially abalone, butterfish, salmon, mackerel, eel, herring, sardines, anchovies, perch, trout and other fatty fish)

shellfish (especially clams, crab, mussels, oysters

eggs

soy products (tofu, tempeh, soy milk, miso soup, soy cheese, soy yogurt)

)cheese and yogurt (goat's milk is best)

Nuts, Seeds, and Cooking Oils

Note: All nuts and seeds (except peanuts) and all high-quality, fresh, unprocessed oils are beneficial for yin deficiency; always use fresh. Oils should be cold or expeller-pressed and organic.

almonds

black sesame seeds (especially beneficial)

canola oil

flaxseeds

hemp seeds

olive oil

pine nuts

pumpkin seeds

safflower and sunflower seed oils, high oleic

sesame oil/toasted sesame oil

sesame seeds

sunflower seeds

walnuts

Cooking Techniques

Note: Always incorporate some fat or oil.

boil

braise

poach

sauté

simmer

steam

Activities

gardening

meditating

practicing yoga or T'ai chi

reading

relaxing/time off work

stretching

walking in a lush, green environment or near water

Foods and Beverages to Minimize

alcohol

chocolate

coffee

excess spicy food

excess bitter food

French fries, chips, and other fried foods

margarine, shortening, and other hydrogenated vegetable oils

poor quality or old oils

refined sugars

Activities and Situations to Avoid

anger-provoking situations and people

anxiety- or stress-provoking situations
and people

dry, centrally-heated or cooled buildings

exercise on hot days

frustrating situations and people

irregular eating patterns

working long hours

overuse of dry sauna

smoking

too many children or abortions (for women)

too much exercise

too much sex (for men)

too much time at computer or in front of
other video display

---

29. Paul Pitchford, *Healing with Whole Foods*. Berkeley, CA; North Atlantic Books, 1993.
30. Maciocia, Giovanni, *The Foundations of Chinese Medicine*. London: Churchill Livingstone, 1995.

8

WET AND HEAVY:
TREATING A DAMP PATTERN

Mary Anne is out of breath after climbing just a few steps to my office door. She collapses her large, fleshy body into a chair, allowing her wheezing and labored breathing to return to normal before speaking. Perspiration glistens on her puffy, flushed face. This forty-seven-year old seamstress was seventy-five pounds overweight when she first came to see me. She put on the weight slowly, beginning when her children were born over fifteen years ago. Excess fat and fluids bloat her abdomen and chest. The accumulation of fluids creates a feeling of heaviness, especially in her legs, hips, and thighs.

Physical activity, including walking, leaves Mary Anne breathless and tired. Just getting out of a chair seems too much effort. "It's so hard for me to exercise," Mary Anne tells me, shaking her head. When she does exercise, her sinuses become congested, her throat collects phlegm, and it is difficult to breathe. Springtime hay fever is particularly a problem, leaving Mary Anne with congestion in her sinuses, a runny nose, and itchy eyes. She also finds herself particularly uncomfortable on damp, humid, or foggy days.

Losing weight has been a lifelong struggle for Mary Anne, despite her efforts to eat low-fat foods. Eating a starchy meal, such as pasta, or something too salty leaves Mary Anne bloated and feeling even heavier and more full than before. Even when she can stick with a weight loss diet, the fat is painfully slow in coming off. With fatigue a big part of her life, Mary Anne often reaches for a bowl of cereal and skim milk, bagels, or toast instead of preparing meals. She keeps her fat intake down by using non-fat milk and yogurt. Thinking they are healthier than meats, Mary Anne frequently chooses pasta dishes and breads instead.

Mary Anne tends toward a pattern of dampness. By reducing her heavy intake of damp-producing foods and adding drying foods, plus beginning a light aerobic exercise program, Mary Anne was able to lose the excess weight and fluids and clear her sinuses. Her legs feel lighter and energized, and her lung capacity is normal, allowing her to feel comfortable walking. She no longer retains fluids in her tissues, and she has more energy.

SIGNS OF A DAMP PATTERN

In general, signs of dampness include fatigue and sluggishness, a heavy feeling in the body, mental fog, excess weight, and water retention. Signs of dampness can also occur in specific areas of the body—excess mucous, or phlegm, a yin fluid, can appear in the lungs, digestive system, intestines, sinuses, urinary tract, or reproductive systems. Bacterial viruses are more likely to become a problem when dampness is present. Chronic yeast infections, urinary tract infections, hay fever, and bloating, although different conditions with seemingly different origins in Western medicine, are all signs of dampness—so are masses, growths, and tumors. Dampness can also make you feel as if you're "stuck" in life. This soggy, wet pattern can be accompanied by signs of heat or of cold.

The most yin of all patterns is dampness combined with cold. People with such a condition frequently feel cold and have a strong dislike for cold, damp climates. Their energy is usually low, and they dread exercise. Their metabolisms may slow to a crawl, and some find it extremely difficult to maintain normal weight. They have a tendency toward apathy and depression. The Western diagnosis of such a pattern may be low thyroid function: Hypothyroid is characterized by many of the same signs as dampness, including feeling cold, weight gain, fatigue, and edema (fluid retention). With dampness and cold, one's circulation is diminished, and muscles and joints may become stiff, sore, and swollen. A feeling of stuffiness often settles into the chest. If you have such a pattern, you may also experience loose stool; thin, clear, or white sinus mucus; and, if you're a woman, urinary tract infections and thin, clear, or white vaginal discharges. You probably have cravings for sugar, alcohol, spicy foods, and warm foods in general. The fatigue associated with dampness makes it difficult for you to find the motivation to exercise, further exacerbating the condition.

When dampness is combined with heat, one has a feeling of being too warm along with emotional symptoms of impatience, irritability, and anger. If you have a damp-heat signs, you may have red, painful swellings somewhere in your body, including fever blisters, herpes, eczema, or other red, inflamed sores, abdominal bloating and distension with foul-smelling gas, blood or mucous in stools, and dark urine. Red rashes, acne, bodily swellings, varicose veins, gastric inflammation, and sometimes hemorrhoids can be signs of damp-heat. With damp heat, mucous is often thick and yellow in color, appearing anywhere from the sinuses to the urinary or reproductive tract. Damp-heat can also lead to bladder infections, including burning upon urination; high cholesterol with plaque-clogged arteries; headaches and mental fogginess; and stomach ulcers.

THE SPLEEN/PANCREAS' ROLE IN A DAMP PATTERN

Dampness—whether with heat or with cold—is associated with the earth element and the late summer season. Although not a recognized separate season in the West, the late summer is a time of ripening and harvest. It is a pause between birth and growth and decay and death, a time of enjoyment and plenty. Appropriately enough, the organ associated with this season is the Chinese spleen, or spleen/pancreas, along with the stomach, which together comprise the process of digestion in TCM.

As discussed in chapter three, the spleen is considered to be the fulcrum of the body's organ functions in Chinese medicine. According to TCM, the spleen turns food into Qi, our vital energy. This energy gives us our vitality and holds our organs and tissues firm and in place—sagging skin and prolapsed organs indicate a weakness in the spleen function. The spleen also regulates metabolism, affecting our muscles, flesh, and moisture. The spleen is what transforms our food into blood and tissue. This digestive function is also said to "control blood," that is, by keeping blood in the vessels. Signs of abnormal blood movement, such as varicose veins and easy bruising, indicate spleen weakness.

Too much flesh or accumulated fluids in the tissues reflects the spleen's inability to handle the food provided and to control appetite. Being too fat or too thin are both signs of weakened spleen function. It is the spleen, according to TCM, that is most directly impacted by diet. For an in-depth discussion of the spleen function, see chapter three.

ARE YOU SUSCEPTIBLE TO A DAMP PATTERN?

Dampness, like other patterns of imbalance, is associated with a particular element and time of year. The spleen and stomach, and thus dampness, are associated with earth and earth-type people.

When balanced, the earth type is nurturing, supportive, and relaxed. He or she is sociable and likes being involved. The earth element likes harmony and peace. The earth element type is generally the one making the meals and enjoys being around food—possibly because food is from the earth. Someone who is an earth-element archetype is more likely to become overweight and suffer from bloating and other signs of dampness than those of other elements. The earth-element type is the one who complains about a slow metabolism. She tends to be round and on the thick side, with large, round muscles. The skin of an earth type is soft, smooth, and peachy. When balanced, her lips are rosy and full.

When unbalanced, the earth-element type's lips become chapped, cracked, and pale. Muscles lose tone. When this type eats too many damp food he may feel sticky, swollen, and heavy. He or she also tends to form lumps and masses, which are accumulations of dampness in the body. These masses often appear in the reproductive tract or the breasts, but they can occur anywhere in the body. Other symptoms include varicose veins, easy bruising, or prolapse of the stomach or intestines. The emotion associated with the spleen and the earth element is worry or anxiety. Just as anger aggravates a liver type, worry weakens the spleen and contributes to digestive problems, including bloating, ulcers, irritable bowel syndrome, colitis, and diarrhea. Even cancer has been correlated with worry. Imbalance in an earth element type is often associated with feeling "stuck" and often frustrated with a job, living situation, or relationship.

DAMP PATTERN				
Element	**Season**	**Organs**	**Emotion**	**Sense Organ**
Earth	Late autumn	Spleen, Pancreas	Worry	Mouth/Taste

SIGNS OF A DAMP PATTERN

Lists are in alphabetical order unless otherwise noted.

Key Characteristics
Note: Listed in order of significance.

feeling of heaviness, often in the lower body

mental fogginess or heaviness in head

excess fat, obesity

fatigue, slow movements

puffiness or fluid retention

masses, tumors, growths

cloudy urine

lack of appetite

Secondary Characteristics

abdominal bloating and fullness

bladder infections

loose stool or mucous in stool

shortness of breath

sinus congestion

sticky taste/feel in mouth

stuffiness in chest

vaginal discharge

Signs of Damp-Heat
Note: The following are in addition to the general damp signs; the most significant characteristics are listed first.

aversion to heat, particularly humid weather

tendency to feel overly warm or hot

dark yellow, cloudy urine

irritable or angry, especially when too hot

headaches

red acne, cysts with yellow discharge, or bumps

desire for cold drinks

gastric irritation or stomach ulcers

high cholesterol, clogged arteries

yellow or dark, sticky nasal, vaginal, or rectal discharges or mucous

burning upon urination, difficulty and urgency with urination (dampness in urinary tract)

Note: The following are in addition to the general damp signs; the most significant characteristics are listed first.

aversion to cold, particularly foggy or damp weather	lack of thirst
tendency to feel chilled or cold	shy, withdrawn
clammy, moist feeling	slow metabolism
clear or white nasal, vaginal, or rectal discharges or mucous	soft, fleshy body type
low thyroid function	tendency to feel depressed
preference for warm, hot, or spicy foods	

CAUSES OF A DAMP PATTERN

Dampness commonly results from poor food choices and eating habits. If you continually overeat, eat late at night, eat while stressed, or include too many damp foods, and especially several damp foods at one meal, you are more likely to weaken your digestion and suffer from a damp pattern. Most importantly, eating an excess of cold or damp foods, including ice cream, pizza, pasta with cheese or cream sauce, cold drinks, and even raw fruits and salads contributes to dampness.

Just as some foods are energetically cold or hot, certain foods are damp. Foods that are cold in temperature slow digestive function and therefore metabolism and our ability to effectively turn food into energy. These foods can lead to a damp-cold pattern. Commonly consumed cold foods and drinks include iced water, iced tea, sodas, ice cream, frozen yogurt, and cold food from the refrigerator. Raw vegetables, sprouts, tofu, cow's milk, fruits, and juices, although not always cold to the touch, are energetically cooling. They have a cooling effect on the body, regardless of their actual temperature and, in excess, lead to a cold pattern and dampness in the digestive system. In his book *Healing with Whole Foods*, Paul Pitchford says "raw foods can weaken one's 'center,' making digestion and assimilation weak." Pitchford explains that the digestive "fire" of the spleen is "extinguished" by an excess of raw food, including salads, raw fruits, sprouts, and juices, causing a watery mucous or dampness.[31] In excess, the cooling nature of these foods leads to dampness in the spleen and eventually to signs of dampness throughout the body.

Too many cow's milk dairy products as well as an excess of raw foods tend to produce damp-cold, whereas an excess of sugary and greasy foods tends to produce damp-heat. French fries, fried meats (including fried chicken), greasy pizza, fatty luncheon meats, margarine, cookies, cake, donuts, and over-processed or overheated fats and oils tend to create damp-heat in the body.

Among the most damp-producing foods are those that combine more than one cold or damp ingredient. Ice cream, for instance, combines both damp-heat and damp-cold properties: The sugar and fat in ice cream are damp and heating, whereas the cold temperature and dairy content give it damp-cold properties. The bottom line is, ice cream is very damp. I tend to observe more damp-cold signs than damp-heat signs in those who overeat ice cream. Let's just say that because of ice cream's ability to not only dampen but also chill the digestive fire, it's one of the worst foods you can eat if you're hoping to lose weight.

Baked goods such as cookies and cakes, which generally combine flour, sugar, and dairy products, and are also poor choices for such damp signs as weight gain, allergies, or bacterial infections. Pizza, lasagna, and other combinations of flour and cheese are also especially damp. These damp-forming foods aggravate yeast infections, hay fever, colds with congestion, bloating, water retention, excess weight, and other mucous-producing conditions.

I sometimes see clients who have reduced their food intake to 1,000 calories or less per day and still can't seem to lose weight. Their diets are generally full of typical "diet" foods: low-fat pasta dishes, non-fat dairy products, fruits, and salads, all damp-producing foods. When they switch to more drying foods, including fish, chicken, rye, and cooked vegetables, they begin to lose weight.

Stress and worry can also lead to congestion, or stagnant Qi, and dampness. In particular, eating while feeling anxious or while working on tedious projects weakens spleen function and sets the stage for dampness. In the Western way of viewing the effects of stress on digestion, energy and blood are diverted from the digestive tract and into skeletal muscles, where it is intended to be used to propel us from physical threat. The stress response is intended to give us the physical resources to enable us to flee or fight dangerous predators. It doesn't serve us so well when we are chronically experiencing and reacting to mental sources of stress such as deadlines and bouncing checks. Too many mental challenges (for example, overworking) and busy lifestyles compromise digestion, especially when we eat while working or worrying about our lives.

Environmental conditions that worsen dampness include damp living conditions, wearing damp clothing, sitting on damp ground, living in a foggy climate, and living in a house with mold. Moldy conditions, in particular, often aggravate yeast infections and sinus mucous and congestion.

REMEDIES FOR A DAMP PATTERN

One of the best things you can do for your weight, digestion, and overall health is to stop worrying. Take a little extra time off work. Relax. Read a book. Take a walk and enjoy the trees and sunshine. Play with your children or your pet.

As you might expect, drying remedies are needed to balance signs of too much dampness. Living in a dry house, preferably in a dry climate, is a big help. Aerobic exercise delivers oxygen to damp tissues and helps dry the dampness associated with excess fat, or obesity, much as the movement of warm air helps dry a wet towel.

Reducing excessive portions at meals and clearing damp foods from the diet is critical. Damp foods to avoid, especially if you have damp-cold, include cow's milk and other dairy products; all wheat flour-containing foods, including pasta, breads, bagels, biscuits, muffins, pancakes, and certain sauces; and refined sugars, especially those found in candy, cake, cookies, and pies. Sinus congestion and hay fever tend to resolve fairly quickly when such damp-producing foods are removed from the diet.

Ideally, to eliminate or prevent dampness and to lose weight, cold foods like ice cream, frozen yogurt, cheeses, foods directly from the refrigerator, and frozen foods should be avoided because they slow digestion and metabolism. Raw fruits and raw vegetables should also be kept to a minimum when damp signs are present.

Iced water, cold sodas, iced tea, juices, and other cold drinks are extremely cooling and dampening to digestion and should be avoided by those with a damp cold pattern. Water and teas are best consumed at room temperature or, even better, hot (best for damp-cold). Cold drinks with ice cubes are an American phenomenon. Other cultures, including those of Western Europe, have long consumed drinks without ice. These cultures show fewer signs of dampness, including less obesity, despite eating fat-rich diets and avoiding gym workouts.

If you have damp-heat signs, you should reduce or eliminate fried foods, including bacon, fried hamburgers, French fries, tempura, potato chips, and deep-fried chicken or fish, as well as foods cooked in poor quality oils (especially fast foods, where cheap oils are often used, and worse yet, reused). Greasy pork sausages, fatty cuts of beef and luncheon meats, lard, and other saturated fat-rich foods should also be reduced, as should all hydrogenated oils, including margarine and shortening. Sugary foods combined with fats, such as donuts, sweet rolls, cookies, cake, and candy bars, are especially bad for anyone with a damp-heat pattern.

Shifting food choices away from breads, cereals, and pasta and more towards cooked vegetables, fish, chicken, and beans is the most beneficial way to resolve all variations of dampness. The best vegetables for reducing signs of dampness include lightly cooked asparagus, arugula, broccoli, broccoli rabe, kale, mustard greens, celery, daikon radish, Napa cabbage, pumpkin, parsley, and snow peas. Many of these vegetables have a diuretic effect. The water and fiber content of most vegetables help rid the body of excess fluids in the tissues, clearing the digestive tract and moving stuck Qi.

Fish, chicken, adzuki beans, and kidney beans are good protein foods for resolving dampness. Signs of damp-cold are easier to remedy with the warming nature of chicken and red-fleshed fish. Signs of damp-heat are better relieved with white-fleshed fish, crab, and beans. Beef, turkey, and pork, however, tend to be damp producing. (Pork is damp and cooling, whereas beef is damp and heating.)

Although an excess of any grain can lead to dampness, some grains, in small amounts, are beneficial. Amaranth, wild rice, blue corn, quinoa, and rye can help resolve dampness. All types of sprouted grains can be helpful to moving stuck Qi and dampness.

Food Combinations and Flavors for a Damp Pattern

If damp signs don't resolve when dairy, wheat, and sugar are eliminated, appropriate food combining can help. As discussed earlier, too many different types of foods eaten at one time affect the tendency of meals to promote dampness. To remedy tenacious cases of dampness, consume protein foods—

meat, fish, poultry, dairy, eggs, beans, seeds, and nuts—at different meals from starches, including bread, rice, potatoes, cereals, grains, crackers, and other high-carbohydrate foods. Vegetables can be included with either protein-rich foods or carbohydrates. The exception to this rule is soup, where a variety of protein foods and starches are cooked together. Chicken-and-rice or bean-and-corn soups, which combine protein and starch, are acceptable for someone with dampness, because they are simmered into one dish.

Fruits are best eaten by themselves. Fruits eaten at the same time as vegetables, sugars, or meats tend to produce dampness more readily than fruits eaten alone as a snack. Fruit-sugar combinations like jam and jellies, pies, and other fruit desserts are particularly damp-producing. By avoiding the combination of protein foods with carbohydrates, you will help digestion to proceed more smoothly. Life is easier on the spleen, and foods can more readily be turned to fuel and energy. Food combining is an excellent strategy for the short term, to improve problems with digestion and dampness. However, once digestion is back in order and functioning properly, food combining isn't necessary.

Stir-fry dishes, grilled foods, barbecued foods, and soups and stews with vegetables and fish or chicken are dishes and cooking techniques that minimize signs of dampness. Cooking with pungent and aromatic herbs and foods also helps to stimulate a sluggish metabolism and to move the experience of "stuckness" often associated with stagnant Qi. Pungent flavorings helpful to stimulating a sluggish digestion include anise seed, coriander seeds, cumin seeds, mustard seeds, caraway seeds, fennel seeds, onions, chives, scallions, ginger, and daikon and other radishes. These pungent foods are considered digestive aids in Western herbology. They aid in releasing digestive enzymes and acids. Cooking with warming seeds such as cumin, coriander, fennel, and caraway can reduce the bloat- and gas-forming potential of some beans and grains.

Overweight people who have signs of cold and dampness benefit in particular from celery seed and fennel seed, along with hot spices, including cayenne, fresh horseradish, chili peppers, garlic, dried ginger, black pepper, and onions.

Those with signs of damp-heat, especially with fluids and fat in the lower part of the body, benefit from bitter greens and other diuretic plant foods, including watercress, arugula, broccoli, and dandelion leaf, as well as mint, and *uva ursi* (made into teas). Watermelon, adzuki beans, cucumbers, and radishes, including daikon radish, are also helpful in relieving signs of damp-heat.

The following lists of foods are limited to those *particularly* helpful to someone with a damp pattern; *they are not comprehensive lists of acceptable foods*. A balanced diet for this pattern includes a broad range of neutral and even slightly moistening choices used appropriately. A few foods beneficial for damp patterns are also listed under remedies for a dry pattern because they are balancing to both. In other words, some foods can both help reduce excess moisture and supply moisture when needed. Only those foods listed under "Foods and Beverages to Minimize" should be eliminated or used only occasionally.

BALANCING REMEDIES FOR A DAMP-HEAT PATTERN

Fruits

Note: Use these sparingly and eat them by themselves as a snack.

apples	lemons, limes
berries, especially cranberries	pears
grapefruit	watermelon (especially the seeds)

Vegetables

Note: All vegetables are beneficial for dampness, with the exceptions of yams and sweet potatoes. The following are particularly helpful for signs of dampness with heat.

alfalfa sprouts	daikon radish
arugula	kohlrab
asparagus	lettuce, especially romaine
bean sprouts	mushrooms
bitter melon	Napa cabbage
bok choy	pumpkin
broccoli	radishes
broccoli rabe	snow peas
cauliflower	squash, summer
celery	turnips
corn (fresh)	watercress
cucumbers	zucchini

Grains

Note: Sprouted grains are particularly beneficial.

amaranth	corn
barley, whole	rye
basmati rice	wild rice
blue corn	

Protein Foods

Note: Listed from most to least drying and cooling.

beans (especially adzuki, great northern, kidney, lima, mung, navy, pinto, and white beans)	egg beaters
lentils	egg whites
peas	goat's milk yogurt or cheese (whole or reduced fat, eaten by itself)
fish, white fleshed	rice milk or cheese
mackerel	

Nuts, Seeds, and Cooking Oils

Note: Always use fresh; use oils sparingly.

canola oil	pumpkin seeds
olive oil	

Foods and Beverages to Minimize

alcohol	lamb
baked foods (muffins, scones, cookies, cakes, sweet rolls, etc.)	nuts, seeds, and oils (for exceptions, see above)
beef	oysters
buckwheat	pearled barley
clams	pork
cold foods, including ice cream, frozen yogurt, sorbet	salt, in excess
cow's milk dairy products (milk, cheese, yogurt)	sugar (sucrose, fructose, barley malt, rice syrup, corn syrup, cooked honey)
fried foods	sweet potatoes, yams
greasy or oily foods	tropical fruits
iced water, iced tea, sodas and other cold beverages	

BALANCING REMEDIES FOR A DAMP-COLD PATTERN

Those with a damp-cold pattern should sip hot teas or hot water throughout the day.

Fruits
Note: Use sparingly.

cherries (cooked)

peaches (cooked)

Vegetables
All cooked vegetable are beneficial for a damp-cold pattern, with the exceptions of yams, sweet potatoes, and potatoes.
The following in their cooked form are particularly helpful for signs of dampness with cold.

arugula

broccoli rabe

brussels sprouts

chives

collard greens

kale

mustard greens

parsley

parsnips

Grains

basmati rice (white or brown)

quinoa

quinoa pasta

sorghum

sprouted grains and breads

Protein Foods

almond cheese (available in health food stores
across the country through Lisonatti in
Oregon 503-652-1988)

black beans

chicken (skinless, white meat)

egg beaters

goat's milk yogurt or cheese

mackerel

prawns

red-fleshed fish (salmon, ahi, trout)

shrimp

tuna (water-packed)

Nuts, Seeds, and Oils
Note: Always use fresh; use sparingly. Oils should be cold or expeller-pressed and organic.

almonds

canola oil

olive oil

pumpkin seeds

toasted sesame seeds

walnuts

Foods and Beverages to Minimize

baked foods (muffins, scones, cookies,
cake sweet rolls, etc.)

pearled barley

cold foods, including ice cream,
frozen yogurt, sorbet

pork

cow's milk dairy products (milk, yogurt,
cheese)

raw vegetables and fruits

cream sauces

refined sugars (sucrose, fructose, barley malt, rice
syrup, corn syrup, cooked honey, etc.)

fried foods

salty foods

greasy or oily foods

sweet rice

iced water, iced tea, sodas, and other
cold beverages

tropical fruits

juices

turkey

peanuts

wheat (white and whole wheat breads, pasta, bagels, etc.)

Cooking Methods for All Damp Patterns

baking

oven roasting

barbecuing

sautéing (limit oil to small amount)

boiling or simmering (as in soups)

steam sautéing (with water or broth)

broiling

stir-frying

grilling (limit oil to small amount)

Tips for All Varieties of Dampness

avoid damp climates

do daily aerobic exercise

build digestive strength (see chapter three)

don't sit on damp ground or wear damp clothing

combine foods properly; avoid protein/starch
combinations; have fruit by itself

eat low-fat soups and stews

---

31. Pitchford, Paul *Healing with Whole Foods*. Berkeley, CA: North Atlantic Books (1993): 304.

9

MOVING AND CHANGING:
TREATING A WIND PATTERN

Elizabeth, a fifty-six-year old administrative assistant, is thin and wiry. She seems almost hyperactive as her body moves in fits and starts. She seems anxious and nervous. Consistent with the tiny abrupt movements of her head and shoulders, her speech comes in sudden, short fragments, as if propelled on gusts of wind. Anxiety and mood swings are common for Elizabeth. Arthritis causes pain in her hands and patches of itchy eczema break out on her arms and belly. She feels worse in the spring, the season associated with wind. Elizabeth shows many of the signs of wind. Her erratic eating and sleep habits only make her feel worse. Her diet, influenced by her English origins, is heavy on fried fish and chips, meats, and rich sauces. She also often skips meals then snacks on chips or cookies.

SIGNS OF A WIND PATTERN

Wind is a moving, changing, yang influence in the body. It often comes on suddenly. Wind can be associated with a pain that moves; it may be an ache in the shoulder for a while, then in the hips, and then, in time, in a knee. Itchy rashes that move from place to place on the skin, tremors, twitching, and dizziness are all signs of wind. Wind blows upward and leads to headaches and dizziness. It may also cause vomiting. Paralysis of any part of the body is a wind condition.

Wind often carries with it cold, heat, or dampness, making it one of the most virulent of the pathogenic factors. Someone with a *wind-cold* pattern has an aversion to cold weather and especially drafts or wind. Waking up one morning with a stuffy head, runny nose, chills, fever, and aching muscles is an example of wind-cold. So is arthritis pain in various joints that gets worse in cold weather. Wind-cold may coincide with exposure to a draft or a cold, windy day.

When wind is combined with heat, one may have an aversion to heat, as well as thirst, agitation and irritability. Too much stress creates heat that can stir up wind. A stroke is an example of *wind-heat,* a condition rising from an overheated liver. The partial paralysis of face muscles with Bell's palsy is an example of wind, often triggered by heat from stress.

The emotion associated with the element wood and thus the liver is anger or impatience. In fact, extremes in all emotions are tied in with liver function, according to TCM, including the emotional extremes of anger and depression in PMS. Excessive irritability, anger, frustration, and impatience are signs that liver Qi has become "stuck" and heat is building. Regularly allowing these feelings to fester further taxes the liver and congests energy.

Certain foods and toxins make matters worse. Old, rancid, or poor-quality oils; hydrogenated fats; fried foods; alcohol; certain medications; recreational drugs; and pesticides all place an additional burden on the liver. Over time, impeded Qi overheats the liver, turning up the intensity and frequency of anger, ultimately leading to shouting, aggression, and sometimes violence. Excessive anger and frustration are among the most damaging influences on the liver. Too much anger, according to age-old Chinese belief systems, aggravates a liver condition, further congesting Qi and creating heat. The frustration of not being able to pursue one's dreams or of feeling "stuck" in a stifling relationship or life situation can tax the liver and contribute to congested Qi. The result is ultimately anger.

The first thing I asked Elizabeth to do was remove the fried foods, hydrogenated vegetable oils, and saturated fats from her diet—no more fried fish or chicken, French fries, or potato chips. She also cut back on red meats as well as sugary cookies, muffins, and cake. Additionally, she began eating cooked green leafy vegetables each day. Greens, especially dandelion greens and broccoli, are therapeutic to the liver. I also urged Elizabeth to develop a regular schedule for meals, exercise, work, and sleep. She began taking more time off work to relax. A multiple vitamin with extra magnesium plus a source of essential fat helped her balance her energy and enabled her to maintain a greater sense of calm. Her family comments that she seems more mellow. Her arthritis pain has lessened, and her eczema is gone.

THE LIVER'S ROLE IN A WIND PATTERN

Wind is associated with the liver, a yang organ. It is also associated with the spring season, a time for new plant growth, and so, appropriately, the element wood. Someone with a wind condition may suffer from spring hay fever, increased joint pain, or a worsening of other wind signs in spring. The liver's yin partner is the gallbladder.

In TCM, the liver is said to maintain the smooth flow of energy, or Qi, throughout the body. Directing life force, or Qi, is no small matter. It is the smooth flow of Qi that facilitates calm, patience, and grace in all we do. When it moves freely and in the proper direction, Qi enables us to progress in our efforts with less struggle and more ease. When Qi is moving as it should, our emotions are balanced and harmonious, digestion is smooth, and our work and projects seem to flow effortlessly around challenges and obstacles.

When the liver suffers imbalance, it can generate wind signs in the body. The physical results may be an itchy rash, sudden irritability, or dizziness. Because the liver also assists the spleen function, someone with a wind pattern may experience problems with digestion, including constipation, bloating, indigestion, gas, and heartburn.

Another role of the liver, according to Chinese medicine, is storing blood. The liver is said to facilitate the flow of blood to the muscles when we're active, to digestion when we've eaten, and back to the liver to restore our energy when we're at rest. When Qi stagnates in the liver, signs of interference with blood movement may include fatigue and release of toxins through the skin, resulting in acne, eczema, psoriasis, and boils. Women may also have irregular blood flow during menses. If the liver isn't doing its job at regulating blood flow, periods may be abnormally light or heavy.

ARE YOU SUSCEPTIBLE TO A WIND PATTERN?

Almost everyone in a fast-paced society, especially when eating fried or greasy foods or drinking alcohol, can show signs of liver congestion along with heat and wind signs, including frustration and impatience. The wood element archetype, however, is more prone to impatience and situations that lead to frustration. Physically, he or she tends to be muscular, with a squarish physique, coarse skin, and strong, slender hands.

At his best, the wood type is confident, assertive, bold, and direct. He or she takes on work projects with vigor, often feeling invincible. The wood type appreciates efficiency, speed, and progress. These qualities apply not only to mental work and career but also to physical activity. Wood archetypes enjoy vigorous physical activity, including bicycling, hiking, running, and weight lifting. Stretching the muscles feels good to a wood type. Intense physical activity and sex provide a sense of relief to the frustration that tends to build in wood types.

The wood archetype is highly susceptible to imbalance from excess work, effort, and stress. When challenged by too much work, he or she can become irritable, rude, edgy, stubborn, and aggressive. Mood swings from anger and elation to depression are not uncommon. When the wood type becomes unbalanced—from too much work, too many deadlines, or a frustrating life situation—he or she becomes impatient, frustrated, irritable, and angry. He or she may develop a volatile emotional state, either dropping into depression and melancholy or becoming angry and irritated.

The wood element type, when unbalanced, also tends to get allergies, especially spring hay fever. He or she may have animal or pollen allergies, which result in sinus problems and itchy eyes. This type may also develop food sensitivities resulting in indigestion, irritable bowel symptoms, or constipation. There is also a tendency to experience headaches, high blood pressure, tendonitis, and painful joints. Women who are wood types are more prone to premenstrual cravings, mood swings, irritability, and menstrual cramping than other types.

The wood type may crave sex or reach for alcohol, sugar, or other mood or mind altering substances, which provide temporary relief through movement of congested Qi. Substances that require detoxification by the liver, including chemicals or pesticides, alcohol, aspirin and other medications, rancid or poor-quality fats, hydrogenated vegetable oils, and excess animal fat, ultimately make the situation worse by further overwhelming the detoxifying function of the liver.

WIND PATTERN				
Element	**Season**	**Organs**	**Emotion**	**Sense Organ**
Wood	Spring	Liver, Gallbladder	Anger, Impatience	Eyes/Sight

SIGNS OF A WIND PATTERN

Note: Most significant traits listed first.

chilliness, aversion to cold weather or wind	head cold with sneezing, sniffling, and coughing
movement of pain or other signs around body	paralysis in any part of the body
itching on skin or in throat	signs of dryness (see chapter seven)
convulsions or seizures	stroke
dizziness	tendon problem
feeling nervous or irritated	tremors, shaking
flu symptoms	vomiting

CAUSES OF A WIND PATTERN

Wind signs might flare on a windy day, with a cold draft, in the spring season, or out of conditions that cause heat. Unfortunately, many of the lifestyle practices and eating habits we cultivate in our modern society lead to wind by impeding the smooth operation of the liver, resulting in imbalance and signs of wind, as well as liver stagnation or liver heat.

The eating habits that contribute to heat (see chapter six) can lead to a wind condition. Greasy, hydrogenated and saturated fat-rich foods can occlude arteries, driving up blood pressure and creating heat. As the heat rises, wind signs may appear as stroke, delirium, or dizziness. A regular diet of fatty meats, cheeseburgers, French fries, chips, bacon, rich sauces, margarine, sugar, and alcohol also tends to congest and overheat the liver. Pesticides and hormones, which accumulate in animal fats, further burden the liver, which has to work harder in order to detoxify the body and circulate Qi. Certain plant foods can also accumulate excessive pesticide residues, when grown inorganically. All vegetables and fruits should be organic; however, spinach, green beans, peppers, strawberries, winter squash, and apples tend to contain the highest pesticide residues.

Along with ingesting such toxins, maintaining a frustrating life situation also fuels wind-heat. The Chinese link between emotions and the liver function dovetails with Western studies of the liver. Research shows an excess of alcohol, drugs, toxins, or an imbalance of hormones, as with PMS, burden the liver's detoxifying abilities, since drugs and hormones must pass through the liver for processing. Clinical and real-life observation show these liver burdens, in excess, can lead to emotional swings, including anger and depression.

REMEDIES FOR A WIND PATTERN

Following a plan that reduces heat signs and signs of dryness generally helps reduce signs of wind that arise from modern day stress on the liver (poor-quality fats, stress, alcohol, toxins, too much work, etc.) Taking sufficient time for relaxation is critical. Avoiding people and situations that cause frustration and anger is also important. Seeking a sense of calm and harmony in one's life stills wind.

If head colds, fever, sneezing and runny nose are frequently a problem, one should take special care in keeping out of cold drafts, heat one's home or office appropriately, and dress adequately on cold days.

Spring, the season that corresponds to wind, is particularly a good time to soothe the liver by eating less food, avoiding alcohol, and focusing more on organic vegetables, especially spring leafy greens. The Western idea is that this helps to cleanse the liver. In TCM, the objective is to sedate and cool the liver. Herbs and acupuncture are effective ways to help clear the liver of wind and heat as well. Making life easier for your liver through diet and taking time to relax facilitates a greater sense of calm and patience. When the liver is clear, the flow of energy, or Qi, throughout the body is smooth and even, leaving an uplifted, content feeling.

To reduce symptoms of wind, cut back on foods that aggravate heat: alcohol, greasy, fried, and fatty foods, saturated fat-rich meats, lamb, excess nuts, cheese-rich sauces, and spicy foods. In addition, foods that can directly aggravate a wind pattern include eggs, crab, and buckwheat.

Meals for a wind pattern should be centered around those foods best for spring: lightly cooked vegetables, especially leafy greens such as broccoli, spinach, bok choy, asparagus, mustards, collard greens, Chinese broccoli, and Napa cabbage; moderate amounts of grains, including rice, wild rice, barley, quinoa, and millet; and, for protein, soy products, legumes, or small amounts of fish or chicken. Meals should be light. Overeating even the healthiest of food congests the liver.

Choosing organic produce and meats as well as low-fat animal products minimizes exposure to liver-stressing toxins, including pesticides, hormones, and antibiotics. These chemicals tend to accumulate in animal fats as well as in certain kinds of produce. Spinach, green beans, winter squash, apples, strawberries, and peaches tend to collect the most pesticide residue. Look for these healthful foods in their organic form.

Foods that can help move a pattern of Qi congestion include watercress, beets, sweet rice, chestnuts, strawberries, cabbage, turnips, cauliflower, broccoli, brussels sprouts, leeks, chives, turmeric, basil, marjoram, fennel, dill, and rosemary. Leeks, chives, and turmeric are warming and should be used in moderation when heat signs are present.

As a rule, if you have an aversion to cold and manifest other cold signs, follow the diet recommendation in chapter five by choosing more warming foods, and avoiding cold foods. If you have an aversion to heat and show other heat signs, choose more cooling foods and avoid hot foods, as suggested in chapter six.

The following lists of foods are limited to those *particularly* helpful to someone with a pattern of wind; *they are not comprehensive lists of acceptable foods*. A balanced diet for this pattern includes a broad range of foods with different properties used appropriately for one's situation. Only those foods listed under "Foods and Beverages to Minimize" should be eliminated or eaten only occasionally. If you have signs of wind plus signs of heat, follow the suggestions in chapter six. If you have signs of wind plus cold, follow the suggestions in chapter five. If you have signs of dampness, follow those suggestions given in chapter eight.

BALANCING REMEDIES FOR A WIND PATTERN

Those with a wind pattern should drink cool (not cold) bottled or purified water.

Fruits

Note: All are okay; see chapters five and six for appropriate warming or cooling choices.
Choose organic whenever possible.

Vegetables

Note: All are okay, but use raw vegetables in moderation. See chapters five and six for appropriate warming or cooling choices. Choose organic whenever possible. The most beneficial type is listed first.

green leafy vegetables (especially brocolli, dandelion greens, asparagus, Napa cabbage)	leeks
beets	parsnips
cabbage family (broccoli, cabbage, cauliflower, kale, brussels sprouts)	turnips
celery	watercress
chestnuts	

Grains

Note: See chapters five and six for appropriate warming or cooling choices. Choose organic whenever possible.

barley	quinoa
millet	sweet rice

Protein Foods

Note: The most beneficial type is listed first.

plant protein sources (beans, lentils, peas, soy products—tofu, tempeh, soy cheese, soy yogurt)	shrimp
fish	

Nuts, Seeds, and Oils

Note: See chapters five and six for appropriate warming or cooling choices.

black sesame seeds	flaxseeds/flaxseed oil
coconut (milk or meat)	hemp seeds/hemp seed oil

Foods and Beverages to Minimize

alcohol

animal fats

buckwheat

coffee

crab

eggs

fish likely to harbor toxins (catfish and
other bottom dwellers, shark, swordfish,
farm-raised fish)

French fries, chips, and other fried foods

greasy foods

lard, butter, and other saturated fats

medications

peanuts, peanut butter, pine nuts, walnuts

pesticide residues in animal fat and some produce

poor-quality or hydrogenated vegetable oils

recreational drugs

refined sugars

spicy food

tobacco

Activities and Situations to Avoid

anger-inducing situations

erratic eating, work, or sleep habits

excessive worry

frustrating situations

overeating

overworking

smoking

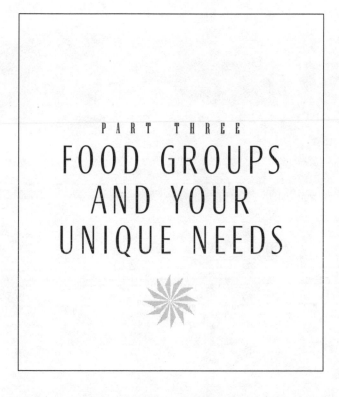

PART THREE

FOOD GROUPS AND YOUR UNIQUE NEEDS

10

PROTEINS:
THE RIGHT TYPE FOR YOU

The Western method of categorizing food (for example, the food pyramid, four food groups, high-protein/low-protein diets) tends to put all protein-rich foods into one category, including poultry, red meats, seafood, eggs, lentils, and soy products. Dairy, nuts, and seeds, while also protein-rich, sometimes wind up in different categories, based on their other nutritional merits. Protein is at the top of the US Government Food Pyramid, which recommends that we include two to three servings of poultry, red meat, fish, or legumes per day, plus another two to three servings protein-rich dairy products per day. These foods provide eleven essential amino acids, the building blocks required for muscle, hormones, immunity, skin, hair, and virtually every other tissue in the body.

According to Western thinking, because all protein foods contain these essential building blocks they should work equally well in maintaining health. If you are protein-deficient, all protein-rich foods are assumed to be equally beneficial in correcting the problem. Popular high-protein diets are centered on these foods, while high-carbohydrate diets eschew them.

While no one argues that we can live entirely without protein, major health claims are made for low-protein and, in particular, meatless diets. Dean Ornish's very low-fat and -protein, high-carbohydrate plan is intended to reverse heart disease and stimulate weight loss.[32] Nathan Pritikin and Dr. John McDougal wrote of similar meatless, high-carbohydrate diets.[33] All these authors argue that optimum health comes from eating a low-fat, low-protein diet based on grains and pasta dishes supplemented with beans and vegetables. The US government's food pyramid also encourages us to eat this way by depicting grains, breads, and other carbohydrate foods as the foundation of a healthy diet, suggesting that we include six to eleven servings each day. Vegetarian or nearly meatless diets, because they are low in animal foods, are also generally low in saturated fats and cholesterol and are thought to reduce high cholesterol levels and blood pressure and thus heart disease and cancer risk, and help control weight. High-meat diets are frequently cited as contributing to these modern-day diseases.

What leaves many confused is that other nutrition authorities purport the path to optimum health requires generous servings of meat, chicken, eggs, and fish, while restricting breads, noodles, and other carbohydrates. Recent diet books, including *Entering the Zone, Sugar Busters*, and *Potatoes Not Prozac*, explain how high-carbohydrate, especially high sugar, diets can lead to weight gain, fatigue, cravings for sweets, and disease by stimulating too much insulin. This fat-storage hormone not only increases the amount of fat stored by your body, it can also raise certain blood fats, putting you at risk of heart disease. Surplus insulin production also leaves your blood-sugar and thus energy levels low. High protein advocates claim obesity and modern diseases can be cured by controlling insulin levels through focusing on meat and other protein-rich foods while cutting back on sugars, breads, cereals, pasta, and other starches. Unfortunately, high-meat diets have been associated with elevated cholesterol levels and heart disease risk, greater risk of kidney disease, and higher rates of cancer.

Many Americans bounce back and forth between high-protein and high-carbohydrate diets. When they grow out of balance through pursuing one extreme, they seek the opposite for a sense of balance. When enough people experience the low blood sugar, fatigue, sugar cravings, and weight gain of the currently popular high-carbohydrate, low-fat diets, the pendulum swings; someone reinvents the high-protein, high-fat plan and provides the "miracle." Those who are tired, bloated, and hungry from eating bagels, Special K™, and spaghetti find immediate energy and vitality from an infusion of chicken, fish, and beef. They need the extra protein for balance after a steady diet of starch. On the other hand, when high-protein diets leave people hungering for bread and pasta, they adopt the latest high-carbohydrate diet, and so it goes.

In our quest for better diets and faster weight loss, we miss the fundamental principle that a balanced approach is ultimately more powerful and effective than are these extremes. The urge to overeat, cravings for chocolate, and excess weight dissipate with balance. With balance, anxiety levels calm down, cholesterol levels normalize, blood pressure drops, and energy levels rise. When you're in a state of balance, you're satisfied physically and emotionally, and your body directs extra energy into burning excess pounds.

The question isn't whether protein foods, as a whole, are "bad" or "good," but rather which ones are best for you and why. After reading this chapter, instead of wondering about whether to eliminate or gorge on protein foods, you will focus on whether you should have the grilled chicken or the filet, the split-pea or the beef-barley soup.

SOURCES OF PROTEIN

Meat and the Case Against Vegetarianism

Tom was seventeen years old when he stopped eating meat. "My girlfriend was a vegetarian, and we both liked the idea of doing things to help the environment," says Tom. At the family dinner table, Tom passed up the roast beef, baked chicken, and meat loaf, instead taking extra helpings of salad, potato, bread, and vegetables. He pushed the meatballs to the side of the spaghetti and took extra slices of garlic bread. For lunch, Tom often ate fast-food fries and burger buns, sandwiched around everything but the burger and washed down with shakes. Sometimes he had bean burritos and chips. Tom always seemed to be hungry and frequently reached for fruit, juices, cookies, brownies, and chips to satisfy his hunger between meals. After two months on his no-meat plan, Tom was besieged with sugar cravings, his energy dropped, and he put on extra weight around his abdomen.

According to TCM, Tom's meatless diet was weakening his *spleen Qi,* or digestion, leaving him susceptible to cravings and fatigue. His emphasis on salads, pasta, fruits, and potatoes created a yin imbalance: too much cold and dampness. While overeating meat may not be so healthy, avoiding it all together can bring on its own set of problems. Meats provide a warming, yang quality that balances the yin foods in our diets, such as salads and fruits. We've built our lives and diets around meat. We've developed ways of preparing our potatoes, vegetables, and breads to balance meat. Pull out the steak and you have an unbalanced meal, one that leaves you feeling unsatisfied because it lacks the *warming* quality of meat to balance the cooling quality of salad and potato. Cultures that use little animal products build their meals around spices, vegetables, and legumes with yang qualities.

Unfortunately, the excess meat, cheese, and butter we've been eating for the past century are clogging our arteries and reshaping us into "apples." In response, many Americans and health "authorities" eschew meat and all other sources of fat—the opposite extreme. By removing all meats and most fat from our diet, the result is imbalance, often showing up as cravings, overeating, and weight gain.

I was a vegetarian for over fifteen years and argued vehemently in favor of a vegetarian diet as the ideal way to human and environmental health. Others follow meatless diets for ethical reasons. Eventually, for me, fatigue, cravings, and other health problems led me to the realization that it may not be so natural to be a total vegetarian. Although some religious groups are vegetarians, few if any cultures avoid meat altogether. "Less than one percent of the world's population voluntarily spurns every type of flesh food. Involuntary rather than voluntary abstinence characterizes the animal food patterns of people in less developed countries," says Marvin Harris in his book *Good To Eat*.[34] Not even the Dalai Lama is a vegetarian, nor reportedly was the Buddha. Following a meat-free, high-carbohydrate diet can leave you hungry after meals, rummaging through cupboards for more to eat.

Meatless eating may deplete Qi, the life force that courses through the body, leaving fatigue, lethargy, depression, and other health problems in its wake. In my nutrition counseling practice, I find that vegetarians have the greatest struggle with flagging energy levels and sugar cravings. Those who eat toast or plain bagels with fruit in the morning are thinking of more bread or bagels by noon. Those who eat tomato sandwiches, salads, or plates of vegetarian pasta for lunch want cookies by early afternoon. What you are missing in small amounts of beef, chicken, or seafood you may be looking for in large servings of bread or cookies. One of the keys to balance is to include just the right amount of animal protein—for you—into a diet rich in vegetables, fruits, grains, legumes, seeds, and nuts. For some people, that might mean only a tiny serving of meat, perhaps only every few days.

For most people, eating some (albeit in some cases very small amounts) seafood, poultry, red meat, or eggs is essential to creating satisfaction and balance. Too much and, sure, you'll probably get fat, burden your kidneys, and drive up your cholesterol level, but too little and you may be left unsatisfied. Balance is like a magic window; when you don't get enough fats, carbohydrates, proteins, sleep, exercise, rest, and so on, you may wind up with disease, out-of-control appetite, and weight gain, just as you would if you got too much of those things. The power lies in that window, the middle path, where you find optimum health, energy, ideal weight, and a deep feeling of satisfaction.

Soybeans and Soybean Products

The yin, cooling, moistening effects of soybeans render them among the most therapeutic foods for yang conditions of excess heat. Both Chinese and Western doctors recognize the benefits of soy in treating and preventing heart disease, diabetes, certain cancers, and menopause symptoms—interestingly, all yang conditions associated with our high-stress modern lifestyles and overuse of alcohol, meats, tobacco, fried foods, and other heating substances.

The health benefits of soy are attributed to specific phytochemicals, according to Western researchers, yet the health effects of soy are much the same according to both Eastern and Western observations. Scientists, who have no means of measuring the cooling or heating properties of foods, have isolated beneficial chemicals (called isoflavones) such as genistein and daidzein, both antioxidants, as well as plant estrogens. These plant chemicals, and probably other compounds yet to be discovered in soy, are most likely cooling in nature.

Plant chemicals in soy have been shown to lower blood cholesterol levels, including reducing LDL (the bad kind) while leaving HDL (the good kind) alone or even elevating it. Researchers believe HDL helps to carry cholesterol away from the arteries and back to the liver where it can then be removed from the body. Risk of heart disease increases when LDL levels are low and HDL levels are high. Studies also indicate soy protein reduces triglycerides, a blood fat associated with increased risk of heart disease. Soy is thought to work by preventing the intestines from absorbing these fats as well as by increasing the activity of certain enzymes that help convert cholesterol to a form more easily eliminated by the body.[35] Soy's isoflavones also work as antioxidants, preventing cholesterol from turning into a harmful form that collects on artery walls as a result of the process of oxidation.

Eating soy products regularly helps reduce the harmful effects of strong natural estrogens when body levels climb, yet it also stimulates estrogen activity when our natural levels fall. The plant-based estrogen-like compounds in soy appear to confer these benefits. Researchers have observed that the more soy women eat, the lower their incidence of breast cancer, reflecting soy's ability to reduce the effects of excess estrogen; at the same time, the effectiveness of soy products in reducing hot flashes, osteoporosis, and other symptoms of menopause reflects soy's ability to stimulate estrogen activity.

These seemingly paradoxical observations make sense from the perspective of TCM, which views soy as a cooling, moistening yin food. Menopausal hot flashes are a sign of dryness, or deficiency of yin, according to TCM. Several western studies have focused on Japanese women, who consume many times the soy products of American women and are known to experience less hot flashes and other menopause symptoms than low-soy eating populations.[36] Asian women, who suffer far less breast cancer, eat enough soy protein to leave circulating levels of soy's estrogen-like chemicals up to 1,000-fold greater than peak levels of naturally produced estrogen.[37]

A study of Italian women, who like American women don't each much soy, found that after twelve weeks of supplementing their diet with soy protein, their hot flashes were reduced by 45 percent.[38] Western researchers identify the phytoestrogens in soy foods as the protective agent; the Chinese have simply noted the moistening, cooling benefits of eating soy.

Tofu also tends to impart a relaxing, soothing quality during times of stress or on a hot day. When I know I've been working too many hours or too hard or there seem to be more conflicts with people and scheduling appointments than usual, I step up my tofu intake. The cooling, soothing nature of tofu helps reduce the sense of frustration and takes that tense emotional edge off. It's a great substitute for beef or chicken on summer evenings because it cools and soothes the body and mind.

Tofu also helps stabilize blood sugar and thus smoothes out moods and emotions. It can be energizing at lunch if carbohydrates from such foods as rice, bread, and potatoes are kept to a minimum. For calming, afternoon energy, tofu is best cooked with lots of vegetables, especially leafy greens such as broccoli, spinach, asparagus, or Swiss chard.

When to Avoid Soy Products

For those with patterns of weak spleen Qi (poor digestion) or patterns of cold or dampness in the body, soy products, and tofu in particular, may not be so healthy. Soy products, including tofu, soy milk, soy cheese, soy yogurt, and soybeans themselves, are cooling and damp-producing and thus not recommended in those with signs of dampness and cold, including diarrhea, anemia, abdominal bloating, depression, pale complexion, and feeling cold. Recent Western research substantiates this correlation, indicating soy products may interfere with digestion and suppress thyroid function, two Western conditions that correlate with Chinese patterns of cold and dampness.[39]

One of the signs of dampness and cold is indigestion, including gas and loose stools. According to some Western studies, tofu, soybeans, soymilk, textured soy protein, and other unfermented soy products may interfere with digestion by inhibiting the function of a digestive enzyme called trypsin. Beans, which are generally cooling in nature, have substances that inhibit the digestive activity of trypsin. Cooking destroys much of this inhibitor. But soybeans have more inhibitor than other beans, and some is thought to remain even after cooking. Irvin E. Liener, PhD, biochemist from University of Minnesota, says that most soybean products contain 5 to 20 percent of the trypsin activity of raw soybeans.[40] Fermented soy products, including miso soup and tempeh, are considered less cooling in Chinese medicine, and as you might guess, have less tryspin-inhibitor activity and are thus more readily digested.

The other issue is thyroid activity. Situated in the front of the throat, the thyroid gland secretes hormones that control metabolism, including body heat. Many signs of low thyroid are the same as those of a cold pattern: feeling cold, irregular periods, and depression. From a Chinese perspective, part of the problem is a pattern of cold, and cutting back on cooling foods such as soy, is recommended. Excess consumption of soy products are suspected of suppressing thyroid activity. Fermented soy products, including tempeh, miso soup, and soy sauce, appear to be less cooling, with fewer thyroid-inhibiting properties and less trypsin inhibitors than unfermented soy foods such as tofu and soy protein powder. Tofu can also be made less cooling by sautéing it with onions, garlic, ginger, or other warming seasonings.

Eggs

One of my favorite breakfasts is a bowl of steamed rice with a poached egg, soy sauce, and toasted black sesame seeds, a moistening, yin-nurturing, yet also yang-stimulating meal. If you have signs of dryness or cold, eggs can be an excellent remedy. You've probably heard for years the perils of cholesterol in promoting heart disease. But not everyone responds to dietary cholesterol and fat with increased blood levels of cholesterol, and many studies refute the cholesterol–heart disease connection. Cholesterol intake has remained about the same for the past hundred years, yet cardiovascular disease has increased by 300 percent during that same period.[41] Recent studies show egg consumption may have no effect or only slightly raise LDL-cholesterol levels, while actually raising beneficial HDL levels.[42] Cholesterol is needed in all cell membranes and is particularly important for the brain. It is needed for the body to make testosterone and adrenal hormones, for estrogen and fat metabolism, and in brain tissue to prevent senile dementia, including Alzheimer's disease.[43]

More recent research indicates cholesterol is only a problem when it goes "bad," or oxidizes, at which point it can injure artery walls and begin to build up in the form of plaque. A generous intake of vegetables, fruits, and green tea provide antioxidants that protect our arteries from the oxidation of cholesterol and thus its build-up.

Eggs are used in TCM to moisten dryness of the upper body, including for a dry throat and mouth, dry cough, and dry eyes. They are particularly helpful for anemia with signs of dryness. Unfortunately most commercially available eggs are from chickens fed a corn-based diet, rendering their product high in pro-inflammatory omega-6 fat (see fat chapter), a fatty acid which is already in excessive quantities in the American diet. There are now better choices in eggs, including range-free and DHA-enriched omega-3-rich eggs from chickens fed a diet that reduces the ratio of omega-6 to omega-3 fats. These are clearly a better choice than conventional eggs, since omega-3 fats may play a role in reducing the risks of heart disease, diabetes, mood disorders, and even cancer. (See chapter eleven for more about omega-3 fats.) Those with egg allergies, of course, should avoid all eggs. However, a mild sensitivity to eggs may diminish when digestion, or spleen Qi, is strengthened.

Dairy Products

For years now, a powerful dairy industry has paired milk products, rich in protein and calcium, with the image of wholesomeness. However, dairy products are generally beneficial only when used by those with dryness, including weakness and a thin, frail body. In such cases, provided one's digestive system can tolerate them, dairy products can provide a moistening effect. The best forms are plain yogurt and cheese; milk itself is more difficult to digest than these fermented forms, and it may also contribute to heart disease.

Mother's milk is the perfect food for a newborn of the same species. It is richly soothing and nourishing, with all the nutrients in just the right balance to enable an infant to form muscles, bones, organs, and tissues. However, once the infant matures and is weaned, milk may not continue to be the perfect food.

Don't Drink Your Milk is the catchy title of a book by Frank Oski, MD, Director of the Department of Pediatrics at Johns Hopkins University and Physician-in-Chief of Johns Hopkins Children's Center.[44] Oski points out that in children, milk can lead to diarrhea or constipation, anemia, skin rashes, ear infections, and hyperactive behavior. The Physician's Committee for Responsible Medicine advocates the elimination of milk from children's diets, indicating it may be a trigger for juvenile-onset diabetes and cause digestive problems.[45] Oski further cautions that in adults milk may lead to cramps, bloating, diarrhea, skin rashes, anemia, atherosclerosis, and fatigue. Milk may also be tainted with antibiotics, hormones, pesticides, and bacteria.

The majority of the world's population cannot digest milk. Many of my clients find they too experience varying degrees of bloating, diarrhea, gas, and cramping if they drink milk, eat ice cream, or consume other sources of dairy. Once weaned, most people lose the enzyme lactase, which digests the milk-sugar lactose.

In her book *Food and Healing* Annemarie Colbin points out that milk is supposed to be going *out* of a woman's body, not into it.[46] She says women suffer more of the build-up effects of milk than men do, resulting in ovarian tumors, cysts, vaginal discharges, and infections, all signs of dampness. Interestingly, breast cancer rates are lowest in countries where little milk is consumed and highest in countries such as Holland, Denmark, and Switzerland, where milk is ingested in large quantities.[47]

Lactose, the primary sugar in milk, is thought to be one of the key risk factors in heart disease, particularly in men.[48] Epidemiological studies of twenty-four countries have shown milk protein (including that in non-fat milk) has the highest association for heart disease.[49] When the milk-rich Sippy Diet was recommended for ulcer patients in the 1960s, those who followed the high-milk plan had a 2.5 times greater risk of dying from a heart attack.[50]

People who can't tolerate cow's milk often fare better with goat's milk. Goat's milk is less mucous-producing than cow's milk. Goats are generally spared antibiotics and graze freely on a greater variety of leaves and grasses, giving their milk a higher nutrient profile. Also, the structure of goat milk is more similar to human milk than is cow's milk.

There is considerable controversy over the use of antibiotics and hormones in cows, particularly recombinant Bovine Grown Hormone (rBGH), a hormone used to stimulate milk production. Choosing organic milk products at least reduces exposure to these drugs.

Meat and Poultry

Although the meat in our diet has been blamed for our excess intake of saturated fats and cholesterol and displacing valuable nutrients and fiber of vegetables and fruits, meat can actually be a healing food when used appropriately. From an Eastern nutritional standpoint, the warming property of beef, lamb, chicken, and venison make them ideal foods for the chronically cold, kidney-deficient individual. Someone with a cold pattern generally is anemic, from a Western viewpoint. The highly bio-available iron, vitamin B^{12}, and zinc content of meat supplies the missing nutrients to correct most anemic conditions. Western studies show red meat provides a more useable source of iron than vegetable sources.

Meats, just like produce and dairy, should be organic. Non-organically produced meats may contain significant levels of hormones, pesticides, and antibiotics. The fat of animals tends to accumulate pesticides and other toxins. In fact, foods of animal origin are the main sources of pesticides in our diets. Hormones used throughout the beef and poultry industries find their way into everything from our chicken pot pies to our steaks. The effects of ingested hormones on humans may include cancer and inappropriate growth and development in children. Researchers from the Netherlands and France examined supposed non-hormone beef bought from the United States and found 12 percent of the samples contained between one and six different hormones.[51] This finding has resulted in the European Union establishing a ban on imports of US beef. Because lamb is commonly available range-fed and raised without hormones or daily rations of antibiotics, it is a particularly good choice for a chronic cold, weak condition.

All that said, beef, like chicken and fish—in appropriate quantities— stimulates and strengthens spleen energy and thus digestion. Red meat begins to erode health when consumed in excess, especially by those with a pattern of heat. Beef, lamb, and to a lesser degree poultry, are warming. Their warming properties come mainly from their high-fat content, which from a Western perspective contributes to high blood-fat levels and therefore heart disease risk. Meats should be used in moderation or even avoided by those with patterns of damp-heat or heat, especially those at risk of heart disease. White, skinless poultry is the least warming and least fatty of the land animal meats and is the best protein choice after fish and legumes for someone with a heat pattern.

Seafood

I recently spent a weekend at some friends' home in Seattle, Washington. My visit was during the unique, two-week period when the Copper River salmon, a special variety, is available. We purchased a huge, deep red-colored fish, fresh from Pike's Place Market at the water's edge, brought it home, and marinated it with a variety of herbs, spices, and lemon, and then grilled it. The sweet, rich flavor of this dark, succulent meat bathed my taste buds with a stimulating warmth and pleasure that I can only describe as deeply satisfying.

Seafood provides qualities and nutrients you can't get from other foods. A regular intake of seafood may reduce your risk of heart disease and cancer, lessen the inflammatory pain of rheumatoid arthritis and headaches, cure psoriasis, and alleviate PMS symptoms, including menstrual cramps. As is discussed in chapter eleven, regular fatty fish intake may also boost your mood and even out your blood sugar and energy levels.

Much of seafood's benefits come from omega-3 fatty acids—specifically, two fats known as eicosapentaenoic acid (EPA) and docosahexaenoic acid (DHA), which are found most abundantly in fatty fish such as salmon, mackerel, trout, sardines, herring, and other cold water fish. The oils in fish enable the body to make anti-inflammatory chemicals called prostaglandins PGE1 and PGE3. The oils in fish help maintain normal appetite and keep metabolism boosted. They moisten and cool our tissues, preventing diseases correlated with the Chinese signs of dryness, including diabetes, heart disease, and menopause symptoms.

Research indicates omega-3 fats reduce the tendency of blood to clot and therefore cause heart attack. They also reduce triglycerides and cholesterol, particularly LDL, the harmful type, while increasing HDL, the beneficial type, further reducing risk of heart disease. Eating at least one fish meal a week may cut in half the risk of sudden cardiac death in men, according to an eleven-year study with 11,000 men aged forty to eighty-four at Boston's Brigham and Women's Hospital.

Omega-3 fats may also reduce risk of certain cancers, particularly breast cancer. The lower incidence of breast cancer in Chinese and Japanese women is, in part, attributed to their higher intake of fish. Laboratory studies suggest diets rich in omega-3 fats (from fish and certain seeds, as well as olive oil, an omega-9 fat, and low in omega-6 fats (from corn, sunflower, safflower, and other vegetable oils) reduces risk of breast cancer.

Omega-3 fats give us smooth skin, energy, vitality, a sense of balance, and the ability to stay calm, all signs of healthy, balanced yin fluids, according to the Chinese viewpoint. Oil-rich fish contribute to our ability to produce moistening, nurturing yin fluids, including hormones, secretions, skin oils, intestinal lubrication, digestive secretions, menses, and other fluids in the body. Fish oils offset the heating and drying effects of too much stress, alcohol, tobacco, and spicy food. Yet they may also help eliminate excess dampness, including excess fat around our bellies and thighs, high blood-cholesterol levels, and an excess of watery fluids in our tissues.

Analyses of coronary arteries during autopsies show those with highest degree of coronary artery disease have the lowest concentration of DHA.[52] Fat and cholesterol-clogged arteries and triglyceride-rich blood illustrate a pattern of dampness and heat. The Chinese say fish helps balance and reduce this pattern of excess. Again, Western studies agree, showing fish oils reduce triglycerides and cholesterol, as well as the stickiness of blood, an indication of its tendency to form clots (and thus a heart attack).

Rheumatoid arthritis and psoriasis pain and inflammation, other conditions sometimes associated with heat correlate with high levels of inflammatory prostaglandins (naturally produced hormone-like chemicals) found in a diet high in arachidonic acid from meat and dairy. Fish appears to counter the inflammatory effects of acachidonic acid, thereby reducing such signs of heat.

Although generally neutral, fish can be prepared so as to take on cooling or heating properties, making it an excellent food for those who are balanced or who have patterns of either heat or cold. White-fleshed fish, such as sole or halibut, especially when poached or braised in liquid, is cooling and thus perfect for someone with signs of heat, including high cholesterol and blood pressure, redness in the face, a heated temper, and a tendency to feel hot.

Pink- or red-fleshed fish, including red salmon and ahi, are more warming than white-fleshed fish, especially when grilled, broiled, or pan-fried with heating spices such as garlic or ginger. Arthritis is sometimes associated with a cold pattern. Here, the darker-fleshed fish, especially seasoned with ginger and garlic, can work wonders on reducing inflammation and pain. One note of caution: Dr. Andrew Weil, author of 8 *Weeks to Optimum Health* and *Spontaneous Healing*, and many health authorities recommend minimizing certain fish, including swordfish, marlin, shark, and other big ocean fish, as they run a higher risk of being contaminated with toxic metals.

Fish consumption helps reduce dampness, including fluid accumulation in the lungs, digestive system (*spleen*, in TCM) and other tissues. In a twenty-five-year study of people in seven countries suffering from chronic obstructive pulmonary disease (a pattern of dampness in the lungs), regular fish consumption significantly reduced mortality.[53] Fish and fish oils are also excellent for reducing damp patterns that tend to occur in the digestive tract (spleen), including indigestion, mucous-producing inflammatory conditions such as irritable bowel syndrome, colitis, and ulcers.

The damp-fighting, spleen-tonifying property of fish makes it an ideal fat-burning food. Western research falls right in line with age-old Chinese wisdom here. Fish oils stimulate thermogenesis, our metabolism, and ability to burn fat. The Chinese would say fish stimulates the spleen and stomach, which keeps metabolism strong and excess fat burned off. The omega-3 fats in fish help maintain normal appetite and control cravings for fat and sugar, another quality of good spleen function. Omega-3 fats cause the release of a satiety hormone known as CCK. This chemical then travels to the brain, where it delivers the message that you have eaten and are satisfied. Fat-free meals are notorious for leaving us unsatisfied and craving more. The ability of fish to stimulate the spleen and stomach functions, you will recall from chapter three, goes beyond energy and digestion to provide the strength, fortitude, and desire to get things done and accomplish your goals.

Even moods seem to be balanced through fish oil, something not missed by Chinese doctors, who have long credited the yin-nurturing, soothing benefits of omega-3 fats with keeping us calm. When consumed regularly, fish leaves us feeling positive, focused, and emotionally strong and stable. Researchers in one study found patients suffering from manic depression improved after fish-oil therapy.[54] Part of the effect, say researchers, may be due to fish oil's ability to stimulate serotonin, a brain chemical necessary for preventing depression. "The magnitude of the effects [was] very strong," says lead researcher Andre Still, director of the pharmacology research laboratory at Harvard's McLean Hospital. "Fish oil blocked the abnormal signal [in the brain], which we think is present in mania and depression."

Omega-3 fats from fish also help control blood-sugar levels, thus evening out mood swings and energy levels. The oils and nutrients in fish feed and stimulate our brain and ability to think clearly. Japanese students often take fish-oil supplements before exams to improve their mental performance. Western research has recently correlated a high fish-oil intake with a reduction in stress and hostility, signs of excess heat that may lead to other health problems, such as heart attacks. A group of forty-one university students were tracked during the three months up to final exams. Some took fish-oil supplements in the form of DHA and the others were given a placebo. The fish-oil supplemented group did not experience an increase in stress levels before their exams as did the placebo group.[55]

A fish-rich meal is also energizing. As with chicken or lean meats, fish stimulates catecholamines, brain chemicals that maintain alertness and energy. This makes fish a perfect food for lunch, one that will give you energy for the afternoon. To get the most out of this energy-boosting effect, keep your rice, potato, or bread serving small at lunch. For extra energy, have a generous serving of broccoli, spinach, or other leafy green vegetables with your fish.

CHOOSING PROTEIN FOODS FOR WHO YOU ARE

If you were going to follow the US guidelines for protein intake, you would be choosing two to three servings of meat, fish, or poultry per day. That amounts to a total of five to seven ounces of meat daily. If you prefer meatless eating, one egg, a half cup of beans, or two tablespoons of nut butters can substitute for each ounce of meat. In addition, the pyramid suggests we include two to three servings of dairy products per day, adding two to three cups of milk, eight-ounce servings of yogurt, or ounce-and-a-half servings of cheese to our daily protein intake.

The Recommended Daily Allowance suggests 0.8 grams of protein per kilogram body weight. This translates into seventy-two grams of protein for a 200-pound person, fifty-four grams for a 150-pound person, or forty-five grams for a 125-pound body. A chicken breast is about thirty grams of protein, an egg about seven grams. Lean ground beef provides about twenty-five grams of protein per three-and-a-half ounce serving, and one cup cooked dry beans provides about fifteen grams of protein. If you weigh about 150 pounds, having an egg at breakfast, a large bowl of split pea soup for lunch, and a chicken breast for dinner, all your protein needs should be covered.

TCM takes a different view on protein. The Chinese system offers no one-size-fits-all serving suggestions and provides no gram requirements. Rather, it recognizes and draws upon the qualities of different protein foods for different conditions. Every form of protein—be it fish or eggs or beans—works a little differently in the body. Some protein foods are cooling, some heating, some moistening, some drying. Beef, a warming, yang food, is ideal for someone who is generally cold and tends toward anemia (a yin condition). Western authorities recognize beef's benefits in the form of iron, which can correct certain types of anemia. Tofu, a cooling, moistening yin food, is beneficial for women with menopause symptoms, including hot flashes (a yang condition). Current research supports eating tofu for menopause symptoms based on its plant-based estrogen-like compounds, which normalize the body's hormones.

Meat, fish, and poultry, according to TCM theory, have a particularly strengthening effect on digestion, or spleen energy. Unlike protein from beans and peas, animal sources are thought to more strongly stimulate spleen Qi, fostering our ability to be productive, motivated, and effective in bringing our ideas to life. Strong spleen Qi, discussed as digestion in chapter three, helps us bring projects to fruition. Strong spleen Qi fuels the builder in designing and constructing a home, the writer in completing a book, and the entrepreneur in creating a business.

Chapter four shows you how to identify signs and patterns of imbalance in your body, including heat, cold, dryness, dampness, and wind, or combinations such as damp-heat or damp-cold. Once you know your yin/yang balance and whether you have tendencies toward heat or cold, dampness, or dryness, you can choose the types of protein that will best balance who you are.

You can also choose certain protein-rich foods to stimulate energy, others for calm. You can choose one kind of protein to warm your body and another to cool you off. Beans, fish, and tofu will provide greater comfort and ease in summer or during stressful periods. Fattier, yang sources of protein, such as lamb and beef, generate warmth and blood-building properties better for winter.

PROTEIN FOODS TO WARM A COLD PATTERN

If you often feel chilled, have an aversion to cold days, and prefer penetrating sunshine to cool rain, you have signs of a pattern of cold in your body. A cold pattern is also associated with anemia, low thyroid, tendency to feel sad or depressed, fatigue, and difficulty losing weight.

You can develop a pattern of cold from eating too many cooling foods, such as raw fruits, salads, juices, and dairy products, or from inadequate flesh foods. You may develop cold signs as you age or when living in a cold climate. Cold is the pattern of imbalance most associated with a low-protein diet as we know it. Meats and poultry are helpful in stimulating spleen Qi, or digestion, thereby boosting warmth, metabolism, and energy. The strongly warming nature of lamb, beef, and chicken is particularly beneficial to those with a cold pattern. These are the most warming protein foods and indeed the most warming of all foods. Red-fleshed fish, including salmon, ahi tuna, and trout are also helpful. Those with cold signs generally benefit from nuts, including walnuts, almonds, and pine nuts, which tend to be warming.

Although considered healthy foods in general, tofu and other soy products (soy cheese, soy milk, tempeh, soy sauce) are too cooling on a regular basis for someone with a cold pattern. They can make weight loss difficult and increase bloating, gas, indigestion, and feeling chilled. Pork and dairy products, including yogurt, are also extremely cooling.

PROTEIN-RICH SUGGESTIONS FOR A COLD PATTERN

Braised lamb loin with root vegetables (braised in red wine, cloves, cinnamon, and ginger)

Grilled flank steak with caramelized onions

Roast garlic and rosemary-infused chicken, including dark meat

Salmon spread with a layer of your favorite mustard and broiled

Pan sautéed trout with butter and almonds

Stir fried beef and asparagus with black bean sauce

Thai curried chicken with vegetables

Chicken or shrimp fajitas with black beans

Chicken or beef satay with spicy peanut sauce

Grilled veal chop with red wine reduction

PROTEIN FOODS TO COOL A HEAT PATTERN

Signs of an imbalance with excess heat include feeling hot, an aversion to heat, menopause symptoms with hot flashes, thirst, a red face, a big appetite, restlessness, tendency to anger, and canker sores. Diseases associated with heat include diabetes, high cholesterol levels, high blood pressure, and risk of heart attack.

Heat signs can be brought on by stress and overwork as well as excess alcohol intake, tobacco, and overeating in general. Specific foods that can aggravate heat when consumed regularly include fried and greasy foods, refined sugar, and spicy foods, as well as too much red meat, in particular beef and lamb. Remedies for heat include relaxation, eating less, and focusing on cooling and neutral foods while reducing heating foods. Cooling protein alternatives to beef, lamb, and chicken include fish, tofu, and beans.

In general, fish is more cooling than chicken or red meat. White-fleshed fish are more cooling than red-fleshed fish. Raw fish, such as sushi, is more cooling than cooked. Beans, especially soy beans, are more cooling than animal protein sources. Egg whites are cooling, whereas the yolks (the source of fat and cholesterol) are heating. A whole egg is neutral.

Among the most cooling protein foods are clams, soy products (tofu, tempeh, soy milk, soy cheese, and soy yogurt), great northern beans, navy beans, mung beans, kidney beans, cow's milk, and yogurt. White fish and most other seafood are neutral and so also a good alternative to red meat and chicken for those with a pattern of heat. The exceptions are mussels, shrimp, and eel, which are warming. Red-fleshed fish, such as salmon and ahi tuna, also tend to be slightly warmer than white fish.

Clams are the most cooling seafood choice. Manhattan clam chowder, pasta with clams, fresh vegetables, and herbs, and steamed clams all make tasty, cooling summer meals. Clams are also helpful for dryness, including dry skin and hair. Paradoxically, they can also help with dampness when it takes form as mucous or edema.

Several legumes are cooling. Mung beans—tiny, round, dried, green-colored beans—are the most cooling of all protein foods. Mung beans are also moisture-regulating, providing moistness to those who don't have sufficient yin fluids and acting as a diuretic for those who have a fluid excess. Cooked mung beans and their sprouts are particularly helpful for damp-heat signs, including red swellings, boils, an aversion to heat, and fluid retention. They help the liver to detoxify and provide a moistening effect throughout the tissues, making them helpful for a pattern of dryness with signs including thirst, irritability, dry skin, and hard stools. Soups of mung beans are prepared in the heat of summer in China for use as a deep, internal-cooling agent. Mung beans are also used therapeutically in China to treat heat stroke, conjunctivitis, high blood pressure, and dysentery, conditions associated with excess heat in the body. Prepare them by boiling them in water or broth for an hour; add your favorite vegetables in the last five to ten minutes of cooking for a nourishing, cooling vegetable-bean soup.

Fish, shellfish, and beans, are most cooling when prepared as soups or in broth. Fish is particularly cooling when poached or steamed.

PROTEIN-RICH SUGGESTIONS FOR A HEAT PATTERN

Oven-baked flounder Florentine with lemon juice, served on bed of sautéed spinach

Sea bass and snow peas poached in saffron-infused broth

Manhattan clam chowder (tomato based)

Navy bean-vegetable soup

Tofu sautéed with summer squash and sweet corn

Tofu and spinach scramble (scramble soft tofu with spinach and mushrooms in a small amount of canola oil)

Chilled edemame (soy beans)

Crab salad with raw lettuces, blanched asparagus, tomatoes, olive oil, and lemon juice

Chilled, marinated three-bean salad on a bed of romaine lettuce

Ceviche (raw, citrus-marinated white fish with tomatoes) on a bed of greens with sliced avocado

PROTEIN FOODS TO MOISTEN A DRY PATTERN

According to TCM, our ability to produce moistening, nurturing yin fluids, including hormones, secretions, skin oils, intestinal lubrication, digestive secretions, menses, and other fluids in the body, diminishes with age, particularly in women. The heat-producing nature of alcohol, tobacco, and too many spicy foods also contribute to dryness. The signs of depleted yin fluids are constipation, dry skin and hair, irritability, restless sleep, the brittle bones of osteoporosis, and, in women, hot flashes and other menopausal symptoms.

Protein foods particularly helpful in restoring yin fluids are those rich in essential fats. The most nourishing oils, and ones we lack most often in modern society, are omega-3 fatty acids. Omega-3 fatty acids are found in high concentrations in fatty fish such as salmon and mackerel as well as in soy beans and flax and pumpkin seeds. Small amounts of omega-3 fats are also found in oats and dark green leafy vegetables. Other beneficial foods for moistening the body include black beans, eggs, oysters, crab, herring, pork, goat cheese, and goat-milk yogurt. Essential fats and other moistening foods work like coolants in the body. They prevent the heat sensations characteristic of all inflammatory reactions, including arthritis, skin rashes, headaches, and PMS symptoms.

Western research depicts essential fats as feeding a chain of reactions that ultimately lead to specific compounds which are anti-inflammatory in nature, called prostaglandins—specifically, prostaglandin E1 and E3, or PGE1 and PGE3. Essential fats help maintain normal appetite and keep metabolism boosted. Alpha-linolenic acid, an omega-3 oil, and linoleic acid, an omega-6 oil, moisten and cool our tissues, preventing problems correlated with signs of dryness, including diabetes, heart disease, and menopause symptoms. Omega-3 and omega-6 oils can be isolated and taken as supplements to relieve dry skin and itchy rashes such as eczema and psoriasis, to ease PMS symptoms, or to help control diabetes. Chinese doctors employ the moistening properties of essential fat-rich foods, and other yin foods and herbs, to achieve these benefits as well as to soothe anxieties from overwork, quell a heated appetite, relieve the brittleness of bones, and alleviate night sweats.

Good protein-rich sources of omega-3 oils are seafood, including fatty fish such as salmon, herring, mackerel, sardines, and trout. A beneficial meal for someone with signs of dryness and heat, in particular, would be a steamed or poached fish such as salmon, mackerel, or tuna. Smoked trout or lox are also convenient sources of omega-3 fats. Oysters, crab (cooling), and herring are particularly therapeutic for moistening dryness. Oysters are considered beneficial for building blood in Chinese medicine—or treating anemia, in Western nutrition. Sardines are said to stimulate Qi, or vital energy, and strengthen the bones. Mackerel is moistening yet able to dry damp conditions as well.

Pork nourishes the kidney system, increasing its ability to provide the body with moisture. It is recommended for those with nervous energy who tend to be thin and dry. Soups made with pork are good remedies for those with dry coughs and constipation. These qualities make pork a poor choice for those with excess fat, conditions of yellow mucous, and tumors or masses.

Flaxseeds—tiny reddish brown seeds rich in both omega-3 and omega-6 fatty acids—are also rich in protein and fiber. Adding a tablespoon or two of ground seeds to your morning oatmeal or onto vegetables supercharges your meal with good fats, protein, and fiber. Flaxseeds leave you satisfied for a long time after meals. They are helpful in moistening skin and hair, in stimulating fat burning, and in controlling appetite. Black sesame seeds, also high in both protein and fat, build yin fluids and blood and are said to strengthens the kidneys, our source of yin fluids. Pumpkin seeds are rich in nourishing oils and zinc, a mineral important for immunity and healthy skin. These seeds impart a moistening quality through their rich omega-3 fat content. They also nourish the spleen and digestive function and are thought to kill parasites.

PROTEIN-RICH SUGGESTIONS FOR A DRY PATTERN

Butterfish or perch sautéed in olive oil with basil pesto

Poached salmon drizzled with toasted sesame oil and toasted black sesame seeds

Marinated anchovies or sardines with roasted eggplant

Stew with chicken, potatoes, sweet potatoes, and green beans (slow-cooked in chicken broth)

Tofu and spinach stir fry with black bean sauce

Steamed mussels or clams in garlic-infused broth with sourdough bread dipped in olive oil

Burrito with chicken, black beans, vegetables, rice and guacamole on whole wheat tortilla

Grilled pork loin on bed of sautéed Swiss chard

Goat milk cheese and sliced tomato with spelt or kamut bread drizzled with olive oil

Spinach-and-mushroom egg scramble or omelet

PROTEIN FOODS TO DRY A DAMP PATTERN

You may have dampness in your body if you are carrying excess weight or if you retain fluids, feel fatigued and heavy, produce mucous in your sinuses, have hay fever, or experience abdominal bloating. Fluid retained in your legs, hands, or feet and puffiness in your face are also signs of dampness.

When dampness is combined with heat, you may tend to be hot and sweaty, have an aversion to hot and particularly humid days, and tend to be irritable or restless. You may be overweight and have a red face, red inflammations with yellow mucous, yellow or green sinus discharge, infections, fever blisters, or canker sores. When dampness is combined with cold, the signs are feeling cold, fluid retention, abdominal bloating, clear sinus or vaginal discharge, a tendency toward loose stools, and a very slow metabolism, with difficulty losing weight.

Many Americans develop these symptoms because they eat foods that, according to Chinese medicine, create cold and dampness in the digestive system. Salad and raw vegetables, fruits, and juices are considered cold and damp. Eating too many of these foods leads to bloating and gas and ultimately to dampness in other tissues of the body, leading to problems such as weight gain and sinus congestion. Greasy or oily foods, refined sugars, dairy products, and wheat products (including bread, pasta, and bagels) are among the foods that foster dampness elsewhere in the body. Combinations of damp foods are particularly a problem. American favorites include pizza, macaroni and cheese, cheeseburgers, lasagna, and ham and cheese omelets. Other particularly damp food mixes include grilled cheese sandwiches, bagels with cream cheese, and ice cream.

Protein foods that contribute to a pattern of dampness include any fried, greasy, or oily meats, including fried steaks and chicken, greasy hamburgers, bacon, sausage, pepperoni, and corned beef. Greasy and fried meats are extremely damp and are most directly linked to weight gain. Other damp protein foods include all types of pork, turkey, and most nuts. From a TCM perspective, cow's milk products are damp and cold and thus associated with overweight, fatigue, sinus congestion and mucous, abdominal bloating, fluid retention, masses, and tumors. Goat-milk products are less damp-producing and can make good alternatives to cow milk, yogurt, and cheese.

The best way to reduce dampness is to focus on cooked vegetable and bean-rich dishes, drying grains, and moderate amounts of grilled fish and chicken. The best protein sources to focus on are skinless chicken meat (with cold signs), egg whites (with heat signs), fish, peas, beans, and lentils. Beans, especially a small red bean called adzuki bean, are particularly beneficial in balancing dampness.

PROTEIN-RICH SUGGESTIONS FOR A DAMP PATTERN

For Damp-Cold (warming)
Spicy white bean and kale soup (flavor with cumin or chili peppers and black pepper)
Garlic, rosemary, and olive oil-marinated grilled chicken breast (skinless)
Gingered baked salmon
Pepper-crusted grilled ahi tuna
Oven-baked trout with minced parsley, capers, and grilled onions
Stir-fried prawns with black bean sauce
Lean flank steak and bok choy stir fried with garlic

Chicken and winter squash poached in a garlic-ginger broth

Lentils, turnips, and mustard greens simmered in curry sauce

For Damp-Heat (cooling)

Cracked crab with lemon juice and mixed greens with light vinaigrette dressing

Poached halibut with minced olive relish and lemon juice

Lentil-vegetable stew

Tofu, broccoli, and water chestnuts stir fried with tamari sauce and fresh mint leaves

Grilled filet of sole with dill and lemon

Mung bean, rice, and vegetable soup

Hummus dip with rye crackers and/or blanched vegetables

White beans and spring greens cooked in broth and pureed into soup

Adzuki bean and watercress soup (simmer watercress with well-cooked beans in vegetable broth, season
   with sea salt and white pepper)

PROTEIN FOODS TO CALM A WIND PATTERN

A wind pattern of imbalance is generally associated with heat, cold, or dampness. Signs of wind include pain or itchiness that moves around on the body, spasms, tremors, shaking, paralysis, and dizziness. Strokes, seizures, and arthritis may also be associated with wind. The best remedy for balance is to follow the recommendations for heat if there are signs of heat, for cold with cold signs, or for dampness with damp signs. In all cases of wind, however, eggs and crab, both high-protein foods, should be avoided because they contribute to wind. Shrimp, fish, soy products, and beans are beneficial for a wind pattern.

---

32. Ornish, Dean, *Eat More, Weigh Less*. HarperPerennial, 1993.
33. Pritikin, Nathan, *Pritikin Program for Diet and Exercise*. 1991; McDougal, John, MD, *McDougal Plan*, 1985.
34. Harris, Marvin, *Good to Eat*. Simon and Schuster, 1985.
35. Potter, S.M., "Soy Protein and Cardiovascular Disease: The Impact of Bioactive Components in Soy," *Nutrition Reviews* 56(8) (August 1998): 231–35.

36. Seidl, M.M. and D.E. Stewart, "Alternative Treatments for Menopausal Symptoms Systematic Review of Scientific and Lay Literature," *Canadian Family Physician*, 44 (June 1998):1299–1308.

37. Zava, D.T. and G. Duwe, "Estrogenic and anti-proliferative properties of genistein and other flavonoids in human breast cancer cells in vitro." *Nutr Cancer* 27 (1997): 31–40. Ingram D. et al. "Case-control study of phytoestrogens and breast cancer." *Lancet* 350 (1997): 990–94.

38. Albertazzi, Paola, et al. "The Effect of Dietary Soy Supplementation on Hot Flashes," *Obstetrics and Gynecology*, 91(1) (January 1998): 6–11.

39. Divi, Rao L., et al.,"Anti-Thyroid Isoflavones From Soybeans," *Biochemical Pharmacology*, 54 (1997): 1087–96; Osborne, S. E.,"Does Soy Have a Dark Side?" *Natural Health Magazine*, 109 (March 1999).

40. Osborne, S.E., "Does Soy Have a Dark Side?" *Natural Health Magazine*, 133 (March 1999).

41. Erasmus, Udo, "Fats That Heal Fats That Kill," Alive Books, (1993): 221.

42. Tamkins, Theresa, "Study Questions Harmful Effect of Cholesterol in Eggs," *Medical Tribune*, (March 9, 1995).

43, 45. Rogers, Sherry, "Chemical Sensitivity: Breaking the Paralyzing Paradigm: How Knowledge of Chemical Sensitivity Enhances the Treatment of Chronic Disease," *Internal Medicine World Report* 7(8) (1992): 13-41.

46. Colbin, Annemarie, *Food and Healing*, Ballantine, 1996.

47. Siegel, Jacob, M.D., "Milk: Does a Body Bad?" *Cortlandt Forum*, April 1992; 123; 50-23.

48. Ibid.

49. Seely, S. "Diet and Coronary Disease: A Survey of Mortality Rates and Food Consumption," *Med Hypoth* 7 (1981): 907-18.

50. Ibid.

51. "Hormone Bad in the European Union," *Nutrition Week* 29(19) (1999): 8; *New Scientist* 162(2184) (May 1, 1999): 15.

52. Seidelin, Kaj, et al, "N-3 Fatty Acids in Adipose Tissue and Coronary Artery Disease Are Inversely Related," *Am Jr Cl Nutr*, (1992): 55:1117-1119.

53. Tabak, C., et al, "Fruit and Fish Consumption: A Possible Explanation for Population Differences in COPD Mortality," *Eur J Clin Nutr;* (1998): 52:819-825.

54. Reuters, "Fish Oil Capsules Found to Ease Symptoms of Manic Depression," *San Francisco Chronicle; Friday* May 1, 1999: A10.

55. J. of Clin Inves 1996; 97:1129-33.

11

FATS:
FRIENDS AND FOES

Despite our obesity, American is experiencing a new kind of malnutrition: a deficiency of fat. Specifically, a deficiency of *essential fats*, most frequently omega-3 fats but also *poor quality* omega-6 fatty acids, *both considered polyunsaturated fats*. Many Westerners consider fat the major dietary culprit in disease. Indeed, we're told to cut fat at every opportunity. Surveys show that fat ranks at the top of consumers' lists of food and health concerns. The Food Marketing Institute's annual trend survey showed that in 1996, 60 percent of shoppers were more concerned about fat than sugar, chemicals, or any other nutritional factor.[56] In 1997, we had 5,600 reduced-fat foods available to us; the choices are even greater today. We've cut our fat intake from around 40 percent down to 34 percent of calories over the past fifteen years,[57] yet heart disease and cancer rates have stayed steady, diabetes has increased, and obesity rates have nearly tripled.

It is true that some types of fat, especially in large quantities, drive up cholesterol levels, thicken blood, and pack on excess body fat. Certain fats are also associated with increased cancer and heart disease rates and even dementia. But not all fats are created equal. The right kind of fat is critical for the prevention of diabetes, heart disease, arthritis, skin rashes, eczema, depression and other mood disorders, and even obesity.

One of the most common reasons people restrict fat in their diets is to lose weight, yet low-fat diets aren't helping people to slim down. The reason low-fat diets don't ultimately work for weight loss is that *we actually need fat to burn excess fat*. Being overweight isn't always a result of too much fat, nor is it always a calorie issue. I have clients who come to me on 800- to 1,000-calorie-a-day diets and still can't lose weight. TCM views obesity as a condition of dampness and weak spleen Qi, rather than a calorie or fat overdose; when the condition is treated as such, excess weight naturally disappears.

Beverly, a fifty-six-year old client of mine, spent a week at the Pritikin Longevity Center in Southern California. The center offers a spa-like program promoting a very low-fat diet. With the goal of losing weight and reducing her high blood-fat levels, she learned to lower her fat intake to less than 15 percent of calories. That meant no meat, eggs, seeds, oils, fish, nuts, or fat-containing dairy products. After just a few months of following the Pritikin plan, Beverly lost a considerable amount of weight, reduced her cholesterol level, and, at first, saw a surge in her energy. Despite maintaining her practically fat-free diet, however, she couldn't get rid of the last fifteen pounds of excess fat and, in time, her energy levels began to drop. Beverly also felt hungry all the time, often succumbing to cravings for breads, cookies, and cheese. Her skin became dry and her scalp itched and flaked. Beverly wasn't getting enough fat. When she began adding back essential fats to her diet, in the form of seeds and their oils, eggs, and fatty fish, she lost the cravings, her energy returned to normal, her skin took on a new glow, and she lost the extra weight.

Essential fat, in particular omega-3 fat, help us get and stay lean by speeding up the rate at which our bodies burn fat and sugars while controlling our appetite.[58] Good fats don't pack themselves onto thighs and hips, they become structural components of cell walls throughout the body and messengers for vital body reactions. From a Chinese standpoint, they strengthen digestion, or spleen Qi, and thus our ability to turn food into energy. Omega-3 fats, in particular, help the kidneys rid themselves of excess fluids, helping to balance a pattern of dampness characterized by water weight.

Good sources of omega-3 fat, such as flaxseed and hemp seed oils, pumpkin seeds, and cold-water fish, increase metabolism and energy production, both signs of a healthy spleen function. Dieting or restricting *protein or* calories, including fats, slows metabolism and leaves us feeling tired, signs of a weakened spleen. Let's face it, if you're tired, you won't feel much like exercising, and activity is critical to burning fat. Essential fats, particularly the omega-3 type, also help maintain normal appetite and control cravings for fat and sugar, another quality of good spleen function, because they cause the release of a satiety hormone known as CCK. This chemical travels to the brain, where it delivers the message that you have eaten and are satisfied. Fat-free meals, on the other hand, are notorious for leaving us unsatisfied.

Essential fats enable our bodies to produce the right levels of hormones, a balance of skin oils, healthy nerve cells, and strong blood vessels. Good fats provide the foundation for our moist yin fluids and youthful energy, suppleness, and sense of calm. The right fats provide the insulation around our vital organs: Every cell in your body—from those that make up your hair to those of your heart—is surrounded by a moist, fatty layer, called a lipid membrane. Good fats also keep your blood vessels relaxed enough to allow smooth blood flow—without adequate essential fat, blood pressure may be high. Essential fats further protect against heart disease by helping to normalize blood cholesterol and triglyceride levels. They reduce risk of blood clots and abnormal heart rhythms.[59]

Good fats steady our moods, improve our ability to learn, and stimulate mental function. Every cell in your nervous system made up of good fats, and the network of nerve cells that orchestrate moods, mental abilities, and behavior are enveloped and protected by a fatty sheath. Imagine this: The messenger molecules that communicate thoughts and feelings are made up of fats! While the mere idea of a fat-free diet is depressing to many, actually following such a diet can create a true biochemical depression. Studies show people with major clinical depression are deficient in certain essential fats. Bipolar disorder, also known as manic depression, improves with the intake of essential fats (specifically omega-3 fatty acids).[60] Cultures consuming large amounts of omega 3-rich fatty fish have lower rates of depression.[61] The descendants of fish-eating populations such as Scandinavia, Ireland, Scotland, and Wales, as well as coastal Native Americans, often experience signs of omega-3 fat deficiency when they adopt low-fat, especially omega-3

fat-deficient diets. Their gene codes call for a higher than average consumption of omega-3 fats, and when they don't get them from fish, resulting
signs of deficiency may include depression, alcoholism, and fat cravings.

SOURCES OF OMEGA 3-RICH FATS

fatty, cold-water fish

flaxseeds/oil

hemp seeds/oil

walnuts/oil

canola oil

pumpkin seeds

dark green leafy vegetables

free range or DHA Omega-3-enriched eggs

THE LOWDOWN ON BAD FATS

Though we struggle to stay on low-fat diets, Americans crave fat, and usually the wrong kind. The top picks for men are steak, pizza, hamburgers, and
French fries. Women go for sugar plus fat: ice cream, chocolate, cakes, cookies, and other desserts. None of these foods provide essential-fat benefits, and,
in fact, these fat and sugar sources can drive up your need for essential fat.

While some fats may have a good effect on one person and a detrimental
effect on the next, certain fats are bad for any body pattern. These "bad" fats
include oils used for frying, as well as shortening, margarine, saturated fats
(including lard and grease), and *old or overheated* oils. They tend to produce
excess heat *in the body* and the resulting signs of high blood cholesterol,
thickened blood, clotting, hardened arteries, and heart disease.

Too much of these kinds of fats in the diet are linked with the Chinese
notion of dampness and therefore obesity. Dampness also contributes to
stagnation of Qi, our vital energy, increasing risk of tumors and growths,
including cancer. Poor-quality fats are incorporated into cell membranes,
creating weaknesses in cell barriers and allowing unhealthy chemicals to
pass into cells and necessary substances to pass out.

Many well-meaning Americans eat poor-quality, potentially toxic fats that are promoted as healthful. Any oil that has been allowed to sit on the shelf for too long or that has been exposed to too much light or heat may have formed toxic compounds, including peroxides and ozonides. Particularly susceptible to such degeneration are commonly used vegetable oils, including safflower, sunflower, peanut, cottonseed, soy, and walnut oils. These oils are often allowed to sit too long on pantry shelves, exposed to light (especially in clear bottles), and used for cooking—all of which lead to the formation of toxins. High heat, as is used for deep frying, is particularly damaging to oils—the free-radical byproducts are thought to contribute to atherosclerosis, impaired cell respiration, reduced immunity, and cancer.[62]

Omega-6 Polyunsaturated Oils

Although promoted for many years as heart-healthy, our favorite vegetable oils, including safflower, sunflower, corn, soy, and peanut oils, may actually increase risk of heart disease and cancers. While they can lower total cholesterol levels, they also often lower beneficial HDL cholesterol levels. They are highly susceptible to rancidity and the associated formation of toxins. When used for cooking or baking, these oils easily break down, leading to cancer-and-artery-disease promoting compounds.

In general, it is best to use these oils sparingly. If you choose to use them at all, they should be purchased fresh in a cold-pressed, unheated form, kept in your refrigerator, and used only on salads or other foods not intended for cooking. If you've got a bottle of one of these oils that's been sitting in your cupboard shelf for more than three months, get rid of it.

SOURCES OF OMEGA-6 FATS

corn oil	soybean oil
hemp oil	sunflower oil
peanut oil	walnut oil
safflower oil	regular commercial eggs
sesame oil	

Margarine and Other Hydrogenated Oils

For years we've been told saturated fats from animal sources are bad for us: They raise our cholesterol levels, clog our arteries, and lead to increased risk of a heart attack. We're encouraged to replace lard, butter, and beef and pork fat with polyunsaturated fats such as corn and safflower oils. Margarine became a "healthy" alternative to butter because it comes from vegetable oils. Only recently have we discovered that the process of making most margarine and shortenings, called hydrogenation, renders vegetable oils every bit as unhealthy, and probably even more so, than saturated fats. Among the most alarming findings are that hydrogenated fats may raise cholesterol levels, reduce the "good" HDL levels, and increase our need for essential fats. In addition, hydrogenated fats appear to raise insulin levels (another risk factor in heart disease), decrease insulin response (a problem for diabetics), alter cell-membrane function, decrease testosterone, and interfere with pregnancy.

Results from Harvard's Nurses Health Study of 80,000 women showed that each 2 percent increase in hydrogenated fats raised risk of heart disease by a whopping 93 percent. By comparison, for each 5 percent increase in saturated fats—the kind found in meats and butter—risk of coronary disease rose by just 17 percent.[63]

Hydrogenated or partially hydrogenated fats are now incorporated into everything from cookies, crackers, and chips to flour tortillas, salad dressings, and bakery products. Hydrogenation is a process whereby hydrogen molecules are pumped under high pressure and temperature into vegetable oils, rendering the final product virtually imperishable and giving it a smooth, creamy consistency. Put in a few drops of yellow dye and it looks much like sweet butter. This chemical process destroys any essential fats and creates undesirable fats known as trans-fatty acids. Food manufacturers love hydrogenated fats because they don't spoil. Margarine can sit in your refrigerator for years and look like it did the day you bought it. Crackers, cookies, and chips can keep on the grocery store shelf much longer because their fats don't go bad.

From a Chinese perspective, eating hydrogenated fats creates heat signs in the body, including elevated cholesterol, high blood pressure and a tendency toward anger. They actually increase our need for essential fats, leading to many of the signs of a yin deficiency or dryness: dry skin, itchy rashes, headaches, irritability, and high blood pressure.

Cooking Oils

The best oils for cooking are the monounsaturates, including olive, canola, avocado, and peanut (needs to be organic and high quality), or the saturates, including butter, coconut, cocoa butter, and palm-kernel oils. New versions of safflower and sunflower oils called *high oleic* offer the heat- and light-stable properties of monounsaturated fats and so are also appropriate for cooking.

Butter, coconut, and other saturated fats are associated with elevated cholesterol levels and are best used in only very small quantities in those at risk of heart attack. But unlike polyunsaturates, monounsaturated and saturated fats don't lower desirable HDL levels. The monounsaturates, including olive and canola oils, are actually thought to be beneficial to heart health; some studies show they lower cholesterol levels. As with all oils, monounsaturated fats should be used fresh, because they can go rancid, though not as quickly as polyunsaturated oils.

Cottonseed oil, used in many processed foods, deserves special mention. It may cause liver toxicity, destroy enzymes that make essential fatty acids in the body, and cause cancer. Cottonseed oil may also increase risk of infertility, digestive irritability, and shortness of breath.[64]

Good Oils for Cooking

canola	butter*
high oleic safflower or sunflower	coconut*
olive	palm*
sesame	palm kernel*

*Oils and fats that hold up to cooking but in excess may contribute to elevated cholesterol levels and other signs of heat.

Oils That Form Toxins When Heated

corn	walnut
safflower	cottonseed
sunflower	grapeseed
soybean	

ARE YOU ESSENTIAL-FAT DEFICIENT?

The signs of a fat deficiency are virtually the same as the signs the Chinese use to identify a pattern of dryness or a deficiency of kidney yin. When you're eating a very low-fat diet or taking in poor-quality fats, you are more likely to experience dry skin, rheumatoid arthritis, dandruff, itchy skin rashes, high blood pressure, PMS, mood swings, irritability, ADD, and depression. Cuts and injuries are slower to heal. In children, growth and development can be delayed and behavior problems may result from a lack of essential fats. In TCM, the kidney system is the source of growth and development. It is also what supplies us with our moist secretions, internal lubricants, and sexual hormones that enable us to maintain a youthful, pain-free, fluid, and supple body. Our yin aspect includes hormones, skin and scalp oils, saliva, eye fluid, and digestive secretions, all fluids that require the right kind of fat. A pattern of dryness in TCM is an essential-fat deficiency in the Western way of looking at things.

Signs of Essential-Fat Deficiency

dry skin and hair	learning and memory problems
brittle nails	mood swings
cracked heels and calluses	cravings for fats and sugar
dandruff	always hungry, not satisfied after meals
dry eyes	premenstrual syndrome
excessive thirst	fatigue
behavioral changes	weakness
irritability	

Conditions Associated with Essential-Fat Deficiency

ADD/ADHD

allergies

arthritis

blood-sugar disturbances (hypoglycemia, diabetes)

depression

eczema

edema

heart attacks

high blood pressure

high triglycerides

low HDL (good cholesterol)

migraine headaches

Are You Essential-Fat Deficient?

1. Is your skin dry and flaky?
2. Do you have a dry scalp or dandruff?
3. Do you have eczema or another dry, itchy skin condition?
4. Do you suffer from PMS or menstrual cramps?
5. Do you have arthritis?
6. Is your triglyceride level greater than 200?
7. Do you often feel hungry or dissatisfied after meals?
8. Do you crave sugar or fat?
9. Do you have trouble losing weight no matter how much you reduce your fat intake?
10. Do you experience mood swings or energy fluctuations?
11. Do you consume wine, beer, or other alcoholic drinks more than three times a week?
12. Do you eat margarine, shortening, or products made with partially hydrogenated vegetable oil or fried foods regularly?
13. Do you consume soft drinks, cookies, candy, desserts, muffins, sweetened cereals, fruit-flavored yogurt, or other forms of refined sugar (raw, white or brown sugar, fructose, corn syrup, and other syrups or sugars) regularly?

Scoring

If you answered "yes" to any of the first five questions, you have strong signs of an essential-fat deficiency and would most likely benefit by adding good food and supplemental sources of omega-3 fats to your diet.

If you answered "yes" to six or more of these questions, the lack of essential fat in your diet is beginning to cause health problems. Begin by eliminating all sources of hydrogenated fats, fried foods, and old or poor-quality oils. If your blood sugar is high or you have diabetes, take steps to control it. Add fish and fish oils to your diet and supplement with hemp oil or flaxseed oil regularly. Add cooked dark green leafy vegetables and soy products to your diet; snack on pumpkin seeds, sunflower seeds, and walnuts.

If you answered "yes" to questions 3, 4, and 5, you will probably benefit by adding a source of gamma-linolenic acid (GLA) to your diet (evening primrose, borage, or black currant–seed oils).

If you answered "yes" to questions 11, 12, and 13 indicates that poor choices in your diet are increasing your need for essential fats. If you also show signs of deficiency, you will benefit from increasing food and supplemental sources of essential fats and reducing your intake of alcohol, sugars, and hydrogenated fats.

GOOD FATS AND HOW THEY WORK IN THE BODY

For essential fats to do their job, the body needs to transform them into hormone-like substances called prostaglandins. There are two families of prostaglandins; one comes from the omega-6 fats in our diets and other from the omega-3 fats. These different forms of protaglandins have opposing roles. We can ameliorate certain kinds of pain, inflammation, and allergies by shifting the balance of omega-6 to omega-3 fats in our diet.

Prostaglandins are chemical messengers that regulate almost every activity in the body, from the production of hormones to the release of immunity factors. Prostaglandins enable the kidneys to regulate salt and fluid balance in the body. Certain prostaglandins control arthritis pain—some make it worse, others reduce inflammation. They control blood vessel constriction and dilation, thereby controlling blood pressure. Prostaglandins help insulin work effectively and can thus help diabetics. If prostaglandins become unbalanced through inadequate essential-fat intake or an imbalance in fats, health problems can arise.

Prostaglandins are divided into three categories, depending on which fatty acid in food they came from. Series one and two prostaglandins, referred to as PGE1 and PGE2, respectively, come from an omega-6 fat called linoleic acid (LA). LA is found in vegetable oils such as safflower, sunflower, soybean, walnut, and corn oils. When the body is healthy, it converts these oils to gamma-linolenic acid (GLA) and then into two other fatty acids: dihomo-gamma-linolenic acid (DGLA), and arachidonic acid (AA). PGE1 is made from DGLA, and PGE2 is made from AA.

Certain foods can block formation of GLA in the body, resulting in symptoms of essential-fat deficiency. A diet too rich in saturated fats and cholesterol (meat, cheese, and dairy), margarine and other hydrogenated fats, and alcohol can prevent adequate GLA formation, as can inadequate dietary zinc, viral infections, and a high sugar intake. Those with PMS, certain types of arthritis, and eczema, in particular, benefit from the direct addition of GLA-rich supplements such as evening primrose oil, borage oil, and black currant-seed oil.

Producing a lot of PGE1 is good, because it keeps blood cells from clumping together to form artery-blocking clots. It also prevents the release of inflammatory prostaglandins and thus helps conditions such as arthritis, headaches, irritable bowel syndrome, and menstrual cramping. PGE1 also helps the kidneys remove excess sodium and fluid from the body. Although also important for health, PGE2, which is produced from arachidonic acid, can be trouble if produced in excess. Arachidonic acid is found in poultry, meat, standard commercial eggs, and dairy products. Very small amounts are also made by the body from linoleic acid, which comes from omega-6 fat in the diet. When overproduced, PGE2 promotes inflammation. An excess of this particular prostaglandin also increases blood stickiness, or platelet aggregation, and the potential formation of blood clots, which can lead to heart attack or stroke.

A third type of prostaglandin, PGE3, comes from omega-3 fats and, like PGE1, is associated with reducing inflammation. Our ability to produce a balance of prostaglandins and thus ideal digestion, blood pressure, insulin levels, immunity, metabolism, and heart health depends on a steady supply of high quality omega-3 fats from food. Alpha-linolenic acid (LNA), which is in the omega-3 family, is found in canola oil, flaxseeds and flaxseed oil, pumpkin seeds, hemp seeds and hemp oil, as well as walnuts, leafy green vegetables, and soy products. (Some of these are also sources of omega-6 fat.) The other principal omega-3 fatty acids are eicosapentaenoic acid (EPA) and docosahexaenoic acid (DHA), which come from fatty fish such as salmon, mackerel, trout, sardines, herring, and other cold-water fish. Most healthy people have the ability to make EPA and DHA from LNA. If you have been taking flaxseed oil as a supplement but notice little improvement in your essential fat deficiency signs, you may need a source of EPA and DHA oils directly.

Omega-3 Fats

Omega-3 fats give us smooth skin, energy, vitality, a sense of balance, and the ability to stay calm, all signs of healthy, balanced yin fluids. TCM considers these fats to be helpful in treating signs of heat and dryness, including dry skin and skin rashes, arthritis inflammation, and high blood pressure. Omega-3 fats provide a moistening and cooling, yin effect, which balances moods and soothes the inflammation of arthritis, PMS, and irritable bowel syndrome. Western research is also revealing a number of healing benefits to a diet rich in EPA and DHA oils. Numerous double-blind studies show that omega-3 fats from fish oil benefit rheumatoid arthritis by suppressing inflammatory chemicals in the body.[65] They also protect the heart by preventing platelets from sticking together and by reducing high triglyceride and possibly cholesterol levels. By lowering production of PGE2, DHA and EPA reduce elevated blood pressure. Even cancer growth appears to be inhibited with diets rich in these fish oils.[66]

Both of these fish-derived omega-3 fats are abundant in brain cells; in fact, the brain is over 60 percent fat. Eating a diet rich in these oils has been found in a number of studies to enhance mental function and balance moods. Their effect on blood vessels facilitates healthy blood flow to the brain. Several studies have shown patients with major depression are deficient in omega-3 fatty acids or sometimes out of balance with other needed fats.[67] Researchers found patients suffering from manic depression improved significantly after four months of fish-oil therapy. These results may be attributable to fish oil's ability to stimulate serotonin, a brain chemical necessary for preventing depression. According to researchers, the effects were strong. Fish oil was able to block the abnormal signal (in the brain) which is thought to be pesent in depression.[68]

The Chinese have long believed a copious intake of fat-rich fish contributes to balanced, happy moods and intelligence. Interestingly, depression in America has increased in every generation since 1900, while our dietary intake of brain-nourishing fats has declined by 80 percent over the same period.[69]

OMEGA-3 FAMILY AND HIGHEST SOURCES

Alpha-linolenic acid (LNA)

flaxseeds/oil, hemp seeds/oil

canola oil

pumpkin seeds

soybeans and oil

tofu

walnuts

dark green leafy vegetables

Direct Sources of DHA and EPA

bluefish

eel

herring

Greenland halibut

mackerel

salmon

sardines

sturgeon

swordfish

trout

tuna (albacore or bluefin)

oysters

free range or omega-3-enriched eggs

Omega-6 Fats

The omega-6 family includes linoleic acid (LA), found primarily in vegetable oils such as safflower, sunflower, corn, soybean, walnut, and sesame. Note that soybean and walnut are also good sources of omega-3 fats. PGE1 and PGE2 are made from these omega-6 oils. We need anywhere from nine to eighteen grams (or about a tablespoon) of LA from vegetable and seed sources every day for optimum health. We generally get more than this amount without adding any additional oils to our diet, however. In fact, over-use of the highly polyunsaturated oils, including safflower, corn, and sunflower oils, is not recommended because they are associated with increased cancer risk.

Meats, regular eggs, and dairy products can elevate levels of arachidonic acid (AA), an essential yet potentially inflammatory fatty acid that contributes to the troublesome prostaglandin series, PGE2. From a TCM standpoint, AA creates excess heat, the signs of which are inflammation, including arthritis, skin rashes, headaches, and inflammatory bowel conditions, including Crohn's disease. Arachidonic acid is richest in the animal foods that are the most heating, including lamb, followed by beef and then chicken. It is also produced in the body from dairy products, also associated with inflammatory conditions.

Many people take in a surplus of omega-6 fats, often of poor quality, including the inflammatory arachidonic acid, while getting inadequate omega-3 fats. In some cases, omega-6 fats are not converted in the body to their useable form: GLA. Signs this conversion isn't taking place or that there may be a deficiency of high-quality omega-6 fats include PMS in women as well as arthritis and eczema.

The ideal ratio of omega-6 to omega-3 fats is about three to one. Unfortunately, our intake of omega-3 fats has plummeted to one-sixth the level we consumed in the 1850s while our omega-6 intake has risen dramatically. Corn-based feed, which has replaced wild grasses and seeds in the diet of the animals we consume, has increased our omega-6 intake from meat and dairy products while reducing healthy omega-3's from these sources. Wild game, which was more prevalent in our diet 50–100 years ago, provides a richer source of omega-3 fat reflecting, nutrient-rich wild grasses. Today's diet, one rich in vegetable oils, modern meats, and dairy products, with too little fish and seeds, creates a ratio of omega-6 to omega-3 more like ten to one or even thirty to one. Inflammatory health problems, strokes and clot formation, high blood pressure, and artery disease can result from overproduction of the PGE2 series. A generous intake of omega-3 fats reduces the tendency of the body to synthesize PGE2 and its inflammatory, or heating, health consequences.

OMEGA-6 FAMILY AND HIGHEST SOURCES

Linoleic Acid (LA)
   safflower oil
   sunflower oil
   hemp oil
   soybean oil
   walnut oil
   corn oil
   sesame oil
   whole grains
   certain nuts and seeds.

Gamma-linolenic Acid (GLA)
   borage oil
   evening primrose oil
   black currant oil

Arachidonic Acid
   poultry
   red meat (especially lamb)
   dairy products
   eggs (regular commercial)

Regular eggs generally contain high levels of pro-inflammatory omega-6 fats and low levels of the beneficial omega-3 fats: 18 ½ to 1 omega-6 to omega-3. Whenever possible, choose range fed chickens, or better yet DHA-enriched or omega-3-rich eggs (available through Gold Circle Farms in Petaluma, California). Gold Circle Farms sell their eggs in most states in health food stores and in some grocery stores.

Recommended Intake of Essential Fats

High-quality essential fats should make up 6 to 20 percent of your daily calories. This is quite a range, but our needs can vary widely. If you are of a fish-eating, Northerly ancestry such as Scandinavian, Irish, Scottish, Welsh, or coastal Native American, you probably need a direct source of DHA/EPA, plus more of it than the rest of us. You will probably feel best eating deep-water fatty fish such as salmon, trout, mackerel, sardines, or herring three to four times a week. If you dislike fish, DHA and EPA are also available in supplement form. Signs that you need a direct source of DHA and EPA from fish or a supplemental oil include dry skin and hair, fat cravings (for French fries, butter, or other greasy foods), alcohol cravings, and depression.

If you are not of fish-eating ancestry, your body can probably make DHA and EPA from the alpha-linolenic acid (LNA) in flaxseeds, pumpkin seeds, walnuts, soy products, canola oil, and leafy green vegetables, most of which also provide omega-6 fats, or linoleic acid (LA). For most people, adding between two teaspoons to one-and-a-half tablespoons of high quality flaxseed or hemp-seed oil to the diet each day is extremely helpful. These oils impart a rich, delicious flavor when added to hot cooked grains such as rice or oatmeal.

Flaxseeds and their oils are quite rich in omega-3 and low in omega-6 fat, making flax an ideal oil when you first begin to enrich your diet with good fats, since most of us have been getting too little omega-3 and too much omega-6 fat. You will most likely see wonderful results by using flaxseed oil for six to ten months, at which point you will probably need to increase your source of omega-6 fats to balance the high omega-3 component of flaxseeds. Hemp seed oil is one of the few foods with the perfect balance of omega-6 to omega-3 oils; it can be used long term as an excellent essential fat supplement. Or you can add another balanced source of omega-6 and omega-3 fats, such as walnuts, pumpkin seeds, tofu and other soy products, or cold-pressed canola oil, to your diet.

SOURCES OF GOOD FATS

Flaxseeds and Oil

Flax is one of the oldest known cultivated plants and is thought to originate in the Orient. Descriptions of its healing properties can be found in Greek and Roman writings dating to around 650 B.C. Ancient Eastern scriptures say that in order to reach the highest state of contentment and joy, flax must be eaten daily. The tiny, reddish-brown flaxseed is particularly rich in therapeutic, moistening omega-3 oils, along with some omega-6 fats. Flax oil is one of the few oils that provides benefits to almost anyone. (The exceptions are those with a flax allergy, of course, or an extremely hot pattern of imbalance.)

Flaxseed provides the richest source of the omega-3 fat alpha linolenic acid (LNA) of any plant food. Its rich essential-fat content is therapeutic in treating high triglyceride levels, heart disease, blood sugar disorders, cancer, obesity, inflammatory conditions such as arthritis and skin rashes, dry skin, and digestive problems, including constipation. Compounds in flax oil may also play a role in regulating blood pressure, kidney function, and immunity.

The benefits of flaxseeds can be derived by using the fresh oil or by grinding the seeds and sprinkling them on food. Add a tablespoon per day of fresh, unheated oil to a cooked cereal or a salad, pour it over rice or vegetables, or take it right from the spoon. When choosing flaxseed oil, make sure it is fresh and kept cool. Don't heat or cook with flax oil. Like other highly polyunsaturated fats, flaxseed oil is extremely perishable. Too much time on the shelf or exposure to heat, light, or oxygen will oxidize these sensitive fats, rendering them rancid, pungent tasting, and bad for health. Good flaxseed oil should have a pleasant, mild, and nutty flavor. It should stay fresh in your refrigerator up to three or four months.

To obtain the oils from flaxseeds, they must be ground into a meal. When consumed in whole-seed form, they provide a rich source of fiber, but they pass through the digestive tract unbroken and the fat and protein do not get absorbed. Seeds can be effectively ground in a coffee grinder at the time of use, thereby allowing their natural seed husk-coating to keep them fresh. Three tablespoons of flaxseeds provide one tablespoon oil and enough fiber to ease even the most tenacious case of constipation. Adding a source of GLA, or omega-6 fatty acids, is important when using the omega-3 rich flax for longer than six months. Flaxseed oil can be supplemented with borage, evening primrose, or black currant-seed oils, or with sunflower seeds. As with use of any therapeutic unsaturated oil, it's also important to supplement your diet with at least 200 IU's of vitamin E.

Hemp Seeds and Oil

Hemp seeds have provided therapeutic value in traditional Russian and Chinese diets for many years. Yes, it's from the same family as the illegal marijuana leaf known for is mind-altering effects when smoked. Hemp seed, however, has no mind- or mood-altering properties. It's also legal. Hemp seed oil is one of the few oils perfectly balanced in omega-3 and omega-6 fats (in fact, it is the only common seed oil containing GLA). This makes hemp seed oil the most completely balanced and most therapeutic essential-fat supplement. Hemp seed oil has a mild nutty flavor that I enjoy poured over hot cooked cereals or rice. Like flaxseed oil, hemp oil is highly polyun-saturated and thus perishable. It should not be used in cooking nor should it be allowed to sit in your refrigerator for longer than three to four months.

DHA, EPA, and Fish Oils

DHA (docosahexaenoic acid) and EPA (eicosapentaenoic acid) are omega-3 fats found in fish, particularly fatty fish such as salmon, mackerel, herring, anchovies, sardines, albacore tuna, and eel. DHA is one of the prin-cipal fatty acids in the brain. The body can make it in limited quantities, but optimal levels are thought to be possible only through foods and supple-ments. DHA is needed in parts of the brain where there are high levels of electric activity, including the nerve endings where communication takes place. DHA is thought to be helpful in normalizing moods and in promoting optimum mental performance, including memory. Low DHA levels appear to predispose humans to early senility and poor mental function. EPA reduces inflammatory prostaglandins and therefore plays a role in controlling inflammation, immune function, and blood vessel activity. It is found in fish and supplements containing DHA.

Fish-oil supplementation is particularly helpful for allergies, diabetes, depression and mood swings, eczema, high blood pressure, high triglyc-erides, migraine headaches, rheumatoid arthritis, Crohn's disease, and ulcer-ative colitis. It takes ten grams of fish oil to supply three grams or more of DHA plus EPA.

Consuming from seven to ten ounces of fatty fish per week plus a table-spoon of flax, hemp, or other omega-3 rich seed or oil per day will provide adequate omega-3 fats for most healthy people. If fish is not a regular part of the diet or deficiency symptoms persist, therapeutic levels of DHA and EPA can be obtained from capsules, which contain varying amounts of these fats. Supplements may be labeled as a fish oil, an omega-3 oil, or a DHA/EPA supplement. The important thing is the amount of DHA/EPA per capsule. Supplements may provide 300 to over 800 milligrams per capsule. Therapeutic doses range from 1,000 milligrams to over 3,000 milligrams. Consult with a nutrition-oriented physician or a nutritionist to determine the best dose for you. Those with diabetes or on blood-thinning medications should check with their physicians before supplementing with fish oils. Some DHA-enriched/omega-3 rich eggs provide 300 milligrams of DHA and a ratio of omega-6 to omega-3 fat of 3:1, an ideal balance and one far superior to the 18 ½:1 ratio of regular eggs.

GLA-Containing Oils

Evening primrose oil, black currant seed oil, and borage oil are direct sources of gamma linolenic acid (GLA), a fatty acid that converts to PGE1, one of the anti-inflammatory prostaglandins. Supplementation with these oils may be particularly helpful in conditions where the body is inadequately converting omega-6 oils to the active GLA; such conditions include eczema, arthritis, and PMS. Among the factors that may limit the body's ability to produce its own GLA include consuming too many saturated fats, hydrogenated fats, and rancid or overheated oils. In addition, alcohol, tobacco, aspirin and other synthetic drugs, overconsumption of animal products, and a poor diet in general will interfere with GLA production. The suggested intake for GLA is 200 to 360 milligrams per day. It should always be balanced with use of omega-3 oils from fish or flaxseed sources.

Olive Oil

Although not a good source of essential fats, olive oil does offer its own health benefits. Studies show that it improves brain maturation and function in animals deficient in essential fats. As a monounsaturated oil, it helps to lower harmful LDL cholesterol while increasing beneficial HDL cholesterol. This heart-healthy Mediterranean oil has recently been linked with improved brain function. A study published in the journal *Neurology*, by Italian researchers found a high intake of olive oil was associated with enhanced cognitive abilities in an elderly population.[70] One reason may be that olive oil increases the amount of omega-3 fats taken up by our cells.[71] Olive oil is also one of the best oils for cooking because it holds up to heat. The first-grade pressing, or "extra virgin," olive oil may offer superior benefits because it is generally processed with less heat and fewer chemicals. Those with a pattern of dryness particularly benefit from the daily addition of olive oil (between two teaspoons and two table-spoons, depending on how much fat is coming from other sources) or olives (three to ten).

FATS FOR PATTERNS OF IMBALANCE

Warming Fats for a Cold Pattern

A cold pattern is characterized by feeling chilled, a tendency toward depression, apathy, a pale complexion, a soft, fleshy body, and anemia. Balance is enhanced through the addition of more warming foods, which includes most fatty foods. The warming nature of chicken, beef, and lamb, as well as the oils of walnuts, toasted sesame seeds, and almonds is particu-larly beneficial for a cold pattern. In addition, oil-rich pine nuts, walnuts, and almonds are also therapeutic for a pattern of cold. Cold-water ocean or fresh-water fish including salmon, herring, mackerel, trout, and sardines provide warming, metabolism-boosting properties. According to Dr. Yu Min Chen, a Shanghai acupuncturist and OMD practicing in San Francisco, fresh-water fish tend to be more warming than marine fish.

High-fat diets have provided warming, healing benefits for years to popu-lations living in cold regions of the world. Native Indians of the arctic have lived off extremely high-fat diets of fatty fish and whale blubber, with little or no health problems. (Disease only became a problem for these popula-tions when refined foods, sugar, and alcohol were introduced.) Their high-fat diets balanced the harsh cold of their environment. Such high-fat, warming diets, however, aren't for everyone and would not be recommend-ed for those with little need for such warmth.

Balancing a Cold Pattern with Fats
1. Avoid hydrogenated vegetable oils, including margarine, shorten-ing, and products made with them (salad dressings, crackers, cookies, chips, fried foods).
2. Avoid pork fat and soybean oil.

3. Include chicken (dark meat), red meat (except pork, free range or omega-3-enriched eggs), and especially lamb, and fatty, cold-water fish regularly.

4. Use high-quality warming oils: walnut, almond, and toasted sesame.

5. Cook only with canola, olive, toasted sesame, and coconut oils.

6. Supplement with therapeutic oils: flaxseed, hemp seed, and fish oils and/or DHA and EFA oils.

Cooling Fats for a Heat Pattern

High-fat foods, in general, tend to be more warming than cooling. A few oils are neutral. Oils and other fats have nine calories per gram, whereas carbohydrates such as breads and vegetables have less than half that. The higher caloric value of fats translates into more heat produced. Saturated fats, including those found in beef, lamb, and poultry, as well as fried foods, are particularly heating. The heating nature of fats can be very powerful, pushing benefits past the point of therapeutic warmth and into pathogenic patterns of heat. Because Americans are so fond of steaks, roast beef, lamb chops, double-bacon cheeseburgers, and fried chicken, patterns of excess heat are common, along with the correlated risks for heart disease, stroke, diabetes, and cancers.

Although those with heat signs will find relief by reducing overall fat consumption, they also need the unique cooling and calming benefits of some essential fats. The best sources for a heat pattern are small amounts of soybean oil, canola oil, avocados or their oils, and cold-water fish, including salmon, herring, mackerel, and sardines. White-fleshed fish are more cooling than red-colored fish. Vegetable oils to be avoided by those with heat signs include walnut, almond, peanut, coconut, sunflower, and toasted sesame oils.

Therapeutic benefits are also obtained from supplements of high omega-3 fats, including flax, or hemp seeds, as well as DHA and EPA or fish oils. These sources are best when balanced with an omega-6 fat source such as borage, black currant-seed, or evening primrose oil.

Balancing a Heat Pattern with Fats

1. Reduce all fats and oils, especially saturated fats, including lard, butter, fatty meats, cheese, and poultry skin.

2. Avoid hydrogenated vegetable oils, including margarine, shortening, and products made with them (salad dressings, crackers, cookies, chips, fried foods).
3. Avoid all poor-quality oils, including rancid or old oils, and frying oils.
4. Avoid cottonseed, walnut, almond, coconut, and toasted sesame oils.
5. Include cold-water fish several times per week.
6. Use small amounts of neutral oils in cooking: olive, canola, or high oleic safflower oils (soybean for uncooked dishes such as salads).
7. Supplement with therapeutic oils: flaxseed, hemp seed, fish oils and/or DHA and EFA oils.

Moistening Fats for a Dry Pattern

Someone with a dry pattern, including fluctuating blood-sugar levels and the inevitable energy highs and lows, will probably benefit from higher intakes of omega-3 and monounsaturated fats such as olive and sesame oils. These moistening fats soothe the hot, dry symptoms in someone with yin deficiency. They even out the delivery of carbohydrates to the blood, thereby helping to maintain healthy blood-sugar levels, normal appetite, and relief from sugar cravings. The right fats soothe a hot, dry body pattern. Fat also nourishes dry skin and hair and mucous membranes.

As with other patterns, avoiding "bad" fats, including margarine and other hydrogenated fats as well as fried and greasy foods, is important. These fat sources can increase your need for essential fats, thereby increasing symptoms of a dry pattern. Daily fats should include fatty fish and fish oils, flaxseeds and flaxseed oil, hemp oil, olives and olive oil, canola oil, walnuts, pumpkin seeds, sesame seeds, and toasted sesame oil. Other fat-rich foods that benefit a yin deficiency pattern include small amounts of butter or clarified butter (ghee), black sesame seeds, omega-3-enriched eggs, whole-milk goat yogurt or goat cheese, and avocado.

If you have signs of a dry pattern, you'll find a supplement of essential fat is particularly beneficial. Good sources include a tablespoon or two per day of flax-, pumpkin-, or hemp seed oil. Other beneficial oils that combine these omega-3 rich fatty acids with GLA-rich oils (evening primrose, borage, or black currant seed oils) include The Total EFA™ and The Essential

Woman,™ excellent GLA and omega-3 fat rich products currently available. More than a tablespoon per day may be needed to remedy some deficiency conditions. Remember to take at least 200 IU of vitamin E when using these or other unsaturated oils.

Balancing a Dry Pattern with Fats
1. Avoid hydrogenated vegetable oils, including margarine, shortening, and products made with them (salad dressings, crackers, cookies, chips, fried foods).
2. Avoid all poor-quality oils, including rancid or old oils, cottonseed oil, and frying oils.
3. Include fats daily, especially from olives, almonds, walnuts, black sesame seeds, toasted or untoasted sesame oil, cold-water fatty fish, free range or omega-3-enriched eggs, goat cheese or whole goat's milk yogurt, and avocado.
4. Use neutral oils in cooking: olive, canola, unheated or high oleic safflower oils.
5. Supplement with appropriate therapeutic oils: flaxseed, hemp seed, fish oils and/or DHA and EFA oils, evening primrose oil, borage oil, or black currant seed oil.

Fats for a Damp Pattern

Any fat, in excess, can contribute to dampness, including weight gain, sinus congestion, vaginal infections with discharge, masses, and tumors. Greasy or fried foods, hydrogenated fats (shortening and margarine), and fatty cuts of meat are generally the worst offenders. Pork fat and dairy fat are also damp-promoting, with ice cream (a combination of dairy fat, sugar, and cold temperature) particularly damp-producing. Fats beneficial for a damp condition include omega-3 fats from cold-water fish plus flax, pumpkin, and hemp seeds.

Balancing a Damp Pattern with Fats
1. Reduce all fats and oils, especially saturated fats, including lard, butter, fatty meats, pork fat, cheese, and poultry skin.

2. Avoid hydrogenated vegetable oils, including margarine, shortening, and products made with them (salad dressings, crackers, cookies, chips, fried foods).

3. Avoid all poor quality oils, including rancid or old oils and frying oils.

4. Avoid coconut and other tropical oils, cottonseed, corn, sunflower, safflower, and soybean oils.

5. Use small amounts of neutral oils in cooking: olive, canola, or high oleic safflower oils.

6. Snack on pumpkin seeds.

7. If you show any signs of essential-fat deficiency, supplement with therapeutic oils: flaxseed, hemp seed, fish oils and/or DHA and EFA oils.

Balancing a Wind Pattern

Follow the suggestions under recommendations for a heat, dry, or cold pattern, depending on your signs.

56,57. Schwartz, Nancy, and Susan Rorra, "What Do Consumers Really Think About Dietary Fat?" *J Am Diet Assoc* 97 (1997)(suppl): S73–S75.

58,59. Erasmus, Udo, "Fats That Heal Fats That Kill," Burnaby, BC Canada Alive Books, (1993): 171–72.

60, 61. Stoll A. L., W. E. Severus, M. P. Freeman, S. Rueter, and H. A. Zboyan, "Omega-3 Fatty Acids in Bipolar Disorder," *Arch Gen Psychiatry* 56(5) (May 1999): 407–12.

62,63. Erasmus, Udo, "Fats That Heal Fats That Kill," Burnaby, BC Canada Alive Books, (1993): 114–15.

64. Erasmus, Udo, "Fats That Heal Fats That Kill," Burnaby, BC Canada Alive Books, (1993): 112.

65, 66. James, Michael J., and Leslie Cleland, "Dietary n-3 fatty Acids and Therapy for Rheumatoid Arthritis," *Seminars in Arthritis and Rheumatism* 272 (1997): 85–97.

67. Maes, M., et al. "Lowered Omega-3 Polyunsaturated Fatty Acids in Serum Phospholipids and Cholesterol Esters of Depressed Patients," *Psychiatry Research* 85 (1999): 275–291; Severus, W. E., and B. Ahrens, "Omega-3 Fatty Acids—The Missing Link?" *Arch Gen Psychiatry* 56 (April 1999): 380–81.

68. "Omega-3 Fatty Acids in Bipolar Disorder: A Preliminary Double-Blind, PlaceboControlled," Stoll. A.L., et. al., *Archives of General Psychiatry* (May 1999); 56: 407-412

69. Brody, Jane E., "New Looking at Dieting: Fat Can Be A Friend," *The New York Times*, May 25, 1999.

70. "High Monounsaturated Fatty Acids Intake Protects Against Age-Related Cognitive Decline," Solfrizzi, V. et. al., *Neurology*, (May 1999); 52(1 of 1): 1563–69.

71. Simopoulos, Artemis, MD, and Jo Robinson, "The Omega Diet" HarperPerennial (1999): 42.

12

CARBOHYDRATES:
A COMPLEX ISSUE

Carbohydrates make up soft chewy sourdough bread, your morning cereal, popcorn, Uncle Ben's famous side dish, and spaghetti. They're also in fruit juices, cookies, and candy. The name itself is charged with meaning for many dieters who either eschew them completely or eat them to the exclusion of almost everything else. In Western nutrition, carbohydrates are considered one of the three major macro-nutrients, along with fats and proteins. They make up the most important block in the US government's food pyramid. Many Western nutritionists throw breads, cereals, potatoes, vegetables, fruits, and sweets into one group. Entire books are written about whether to eat more or less of these foods as a whole.

From a TCM point of view, carbohydrate foods don't fit into one category any more than protein foods or fats do. Some carbohydrate-rich foods are cooling and damp, whereas others are warm and drying. That means some types of bread or crackers may leave you feeling bloated and fatigued, whereas others won't cause you to experience these symptoms. Certain starch-rich foods may boost your energy and facilitate a sense of calm; others may leave you tired and restless. Some complex carbohydrates may help you lose excess weight, while others may make it seem impossible.

Just as with fat- and protein-rich foods, carbohydrates need to be selected based on your unique needs. Some people will benefit by increasing their intake of pasta, bread, or other wheat-based carbohydrate foods; others will find health benefits by reducing them. Each carbohydrate food—be it bread, oatmeal, squash, cookies, rice, rye, barley, polenta, apples, or carrots—has a different effect on the body. Once you learn the best choices for your body pattern, you can eat the cereals, pastas, breads, and other foods that facilitate energy, health, and ideal body weight for you.

CHOOSING THE RIGHT CARBOHYDRATES FOR YOU

Chapter four shows you how to identify signs and patterns of imbalance in your body, including heat, cold, dryness, wind, dampness, or combinations such as damp-heat or damp-cold. Once you know your yin/yang balance and whether you have tendencies toward heat or cold,

CARBOHYDRATES MADE SIMPLE

Carbohydrates can be either "simple" or "complex." Whole wheat, oats, barley, and other whole grains, as well as vegetables, are sources of unrefined complex carbohydrates. White flour-based breads and noodles, although refined, are also considered complex carbohydrates. Sucrose, fructose, dextrose, high-fructose corn syrup, maple syrup, and honey are all simple carbohydrates, or sugars, usually refined in some way and incorporated into our favorite cookies, candy, cakes, and muffins. Fruit and milk products, although not refined, also contain simple sugars—fruits contain fructose, glucose, and sucrose, and milk contains lactose.

Unrefined or unprocessed complex carbohydrates are generally more healthful than refined, or simple carbohydrates. First, they come packaged by nature with important vitamins, minerals, and fiber. Second, they are released more slowly into the blood stream than are processed or simple carbohydrates. This slow release of energy puts less of a burden on organs such as the pancreas and adrenals, which have to respond to high blood-sugar levels by releasing hormones that are not needed by the body at that time. A can of cola, which, by the way, contains about ten teaspoons of sugar, drives up blood sugar quickly, causing the pancreas to release insulin and the adrenals to put out adrenaline. When the body is forced to do this regularly, health problems result, including many of those associated with yin deficiency, or dryness: fatigue, blood-sugar imbalances, weak bones, anxiety, and hot flashes. This chapter focuses on complex carbohydrates. For an in-depth discussion of the health problems associated with sugars, see chapter thirteen.

dampness or dryness, you can choose the types of breads, cereals, and other carbohydrates that will best balance who you are. Those with a damp pattern should pay especially careful attention to their wheat (white and whole-wheat flour, breads, and so on), refined sugar, and fruit juice consumption, since these carbohydrates are the main culprits in many damp conditions. Overeating any food can lead to dampness, but excess refined grains (especially wheat, one of the staples of western society), in particular, can cause signs of dampness. Grain-based foods are thus one of the first to go on many weight loss programs. For this reason, the damp pattern is discussed in greater depth here than are the other patterns. In addition to choosing specific carbohydrates to balance your patterns of imbalance, you can also alter your carbohydrate intake for added energy or enhanced calm. You can use certain carbohydrates for warmth, others to cool down.

Carbohydrates for a Damp Pattern

Most carbohydrate-rich foods are yin relative to most protein-rich foods. Thus, they tend to be calming (a yin quality), but they can also be the most damp-producing foods in the Chinese system. Of all the patterns, someone with a pattern of dampness generally has the most health problems on a high-wheat and/or high-sugar diet. Dampness in the spleen, which translates into problems with digestion (bloating), low energy, weight gain, and sinus congestion, is most often linked with breads, pasta, and other wheat-based foods, as well as with refined sugars and the milk-sugar lactose. Gas, mucous, cramping, diarrhea, constipation, and excess weight are often alleviated when people stop eating these foods. To remedy digestive problems, many Western health practitioners recommend a diet based almost exclusively on meats, poultry, fish, beans, and vegetables. But carbohydrates as a whole are not causing the problem; rather, the specific carbohydrate sources most common in our diet—wheat, milk (specifically the milk-sugar, lactose), and refined sugars—are more likely to blame.

The tendency to accumulate excess fat and fluid in your tissues, and mucous in your sinuses, as well as a feeling of fatigue and heaviness—in other words, a damp pattern—is best balanced by a diet low in damp-producing foods. The reason many weight-loss plans advise drastic reductions in carbohydrates is that many carbohydrate foods, and especially wheat, are, according to TCM, damp. Since wheat (breads, pasta, bagels, cereals) is the staple grain in Western diets, it's little wonder we have high obesity rates, sinus problems, and other signs of dampness.

Eating Consciously to Improve Digestion

The way we eat our food plays a role in how dampening it is to our systems. Digestion of carbohydrates begins in the mouth, with an enzyme in saliva called amylase. Carbohydrate foods, and in particular grains, need to be chewed into tiny fragments and to be in contact with amylase for a significant period of time in order to break down the starch molecules into small enough pieces for the digestive system to handle them. If you're in a big hurry and gulp your food with little chewing, you put a burden on your digestive system, increasing the likelihood of fluids being drawn into your stomach, with resulting abdominal bloating and other signs of dampness. A good rule of thumb is to chew every bite, especially grains, from twenty-five to fifty times.

Along with chewing, taking time to relax while eating is important. Many of my clients confess to eating while driving, while shopping, or while reviewing business plans and reports. By focusing on your meal, and not the front-page war story, a TV drama, or the drive to work, you help the digestive process. Relaxing while eating facilitates the release of appropriate digestive secretions to break down your foods, making digestion, the burning of calories, and the liberation of energy a smoother, more effective process. As our society picks up its collective pace, adding more and more activities, we seem to have more problems with digesting grains. Wheat "allergies," which have signs paralleling dampness, are becoming more common (see section below on wheat). Wheat- and gluten-free foods are becoming widely available as an option to whole-wheat and white flour foods. Perhaps by slowing down, chewing our food more thoroughly, and eating more consciously, we can reduce such digestive allergy signs.

Simple Food Combining for Dampness

When digesting grains is still a problem even after you have identified the right grain for your pattern and follow the tips above, simple food combining may reduce indigestion, bloating, and other signs of dampness. The concept of food combination is discussed in detail in chapter eight. The basic idea is to eat breads, rice, pasta, and potatoes at different times from fish, meats, beans, and eggs. Carbohydrates may be consumed with vegetables, other starches or grains, and oil, but not with protein foods. Fruits and dairy products should be eaten by themselves. Some people find practicing simple food combining for one or two meals per day improves digestion and is helpful with weight loss.

One of the more damp food combinations is sugar and starch. The protein-sugar reaction that occurs during baking makes these foods particularly difficult to digest and thus weakening to spleen Qi. That means cookies, muffins, and cake, for instance, are extremely damp-producing foods. Putting jam on your toast or syrup on your pancakes will increase the damp-producing nature of these foods.

Carbohydrates that Reduce Dampness

All grains, including wheat, become less damp-producing when they are sprouted, especially when baked as a bread. Sprouted grains make a delightfully sweet, dense bread called manna or essene bread, which is available in most health food stores. Cooking also leaves grains less damp-producing than they are when raw. Cooked whole grains that reduce a pattern of dampness include amaranth, corn, buckwheat, unrefined barley, rye, wild rice, and basmati rice. Amaranth and whole barley are unique in that they restore moisture to a dry pattern and help rid the body of excess fluids in a damp pattern. Other carbohydrate-rich foods that help reduce signs of dampness include cooked pumpkin, turnips, rye, corn, and small amounts of raw honey.

Carbohydrates for a Cold Pattern

Winter temperatures can chill us to the bone, making it seem impossible to get warm again. Some people always seem to be cold, even when temperatures warm up. Their metabolisms run slow, they gain weight easily, and they often seem depressed or melancholy. Hot, cooked grains, especially when warmed further by the addition of warming spices, are particularly effective in warming our body core and moods.

Although no grains are particularly heating, the grains that provide the most warmth for balance in a cold pattern include oatmeal, buckwheat, kamut, spelt, buckwheat, quinoa, sweet rice, and basmati rice. Someone with a cold pattern benefits most by eating grains that are well cooked and served hot. Oatmeal can be made even more warming with the addition of cinnamon. A savory buckwheat or quinoa side dish can be cooked with sautéed garlic and onions. Fresh or dried ginger offers a delicious way to deepen the warmth of sweet or basmati rice.

In addition, winter vegetables such as parsnips and winter squash also tend to be warming. A winter evening meal might include baked winter squash topped with a light brush of clarified butter and sprinkling of cinnamon.

Carbohydrates for a Heat Pattern

When I first met him, Ron was a sixty-eight-year-old politician, a robust, overweight, loud-spoken, sometimes irritable type. His high cholesterol and blood pressure had his physician and me concerned. For Ron, shifting away from his yang diet of steaks, roast beef, venison, and cocktails toward more pasta, rice, whole-grain breads, vegetables, and other carbohydrate foods restored balance. When he eats rice or pasta and vegetable dishes, he feels calmer, less agitated. After just a few months on this diet, Ron reduced his cholesterol by twenty-five points and his weight by fifteen pounds.

Grain foods, including cereals, pastas, and breads, are generally relatively yin in that they are less heating than meats, eggs and fats. Shifting to more of a grain-based diet from a high-meat diet is helpful in balancing someone with a yang pattern of excess heat. The best grains for a heat pattern are those most cooling and/or moistening, including millet, wheat, spelt, amaranth, wild rice, corn, blue corn, whole barley, and potatoes.

Carbohydrates for a Dry Pattern

When fifty-five-year-old Janet went on a high-protein, low-carbohydrate diet, she cut out all breads and noodles and lost her unwanted weight. She also became anxious and edgy and found it difficult to relax into sleep, signs of dryness. Her sugar cravings became overwhelming. By adding back less damp-producing carbohydrates, including basmati rice, rye, and wild rice, to her evening meal, her energy and moods evened out and she was able to sleep through the night. The added grains provided a moistening and claming quality without contributing to dampness and weight gain. Unlike breads and noodles, the rice choices and rye didn't cause her unwanted pounds to return.

Signs of dryness tend to set in with too much exercise, stress, and age, leaving us with dry skin and hair, irritability, insomnia, sometimes a dry mouth and throat, blood-sugar fluctuations, and often sugar cravings. Menopause symptoms are often signs of dryness, or yin deficiency. The right whole grains can moisten the body, helping to balance blood sugar and calm irritability. They can also keep athletes from developing signs of dryness. The ability of certain whole grains to release carbohydrates slowly into the blood helps keep blood-sugar levels stable, while the yin nature of certain grains soothes and moistens the body.

For most people with a pattern of dryness, helpful moistening grains include kamut, sweet rice, quinoa, millet, whole barley, and spelt, as well as whole wheat, sweet potatoes, and white potatoes. Although white flour in the form of breads and noodles is moistening, it is often too much so. In addition, its tendency to raise insulin levels and cause digestive problems makes it a poor choice for many.

Carbohydrates for a Wind Pattern

As you will recall from chapter nine, a wind pattern can carry with it any of the other patterns of imbalance: heat, cold, dampness, or dryness. If you experience twitching, nervousness, itching, paralysis, seizures, or other signs of wind, follow carbohydrate suggestions for the main pattern most appropriate for you in order to balance your signs. Buckwheat is the only carbohydrate food specifically contraindicated for wind.

Choosing Foods to Stimulate Productivity and Enhance Relaxation

In traditional China, people tend to live at a slower pace than in Western cultures. Their diet, one rich in rice and vegetables, helps facilitate that quality of energy and balance. Each meal balances a hearty serving of rice with a generous portion of vegetables and small to moderate amounts of meat, poultry, fish, or eggs. Choosing this balance between carbohydrate and protein foods allows them to maintain a constant modest quality in their energy levels.

At certain times you may want this balanced sense of calm in your life, while at other times you may want to encourage a burst of activity or the ability to turn off the harried pace of your busy day. Knowing how carbohydrates impact the yin or yang qualities of your brain chemistry and thus your moods enables you to make these moment-to-moment food choices.

For most people, vital, yang energy peaks in the mornings and stays that way through lunchtime. We get the most accomplished in the mornings, when we are the most clear-headed and productive. We're on. After the midday meal, energy levels tend to wane, leaving us sleepy, more apt to make mistakes, or at the very least much more relaxed, a relatively yin state. The yang qualities of alertness and productivity are again revived in the late afternoon. We can consciously choose our carbohydrate and protein foods to impact these fluctuations in energy and productivity, as well as our ability to relax.

Carbohydrate foods, including breads, rice, and other grains, as well as vegetables and fruits, are the yin counterpart to protein foods such as meats and poultry. Carbohydrate-rich meals thus tend to leave us feeling pleasantly relaxed, softer, more receptive, and sometime even sleepy—all relatively yin states. According to MIT researchers, high-carbohydrate foods—such as breads and sweets—produce large amounts of the brain chemical serotonin, which can be sedating in nature. In fact, say researchers, eating a high-carbohydrate snack leaves people relaxed and even sleepy for over three hours.

This seems to be particularly the case with lunch. According to Dr. Judith Wurtman, PhD, a food and mood researcher at MIT, eating a carbohydrate-rich lunch induces a sense of calm, relaxation, dulled mental performance, and sleepiness in the subsequent afternoon hours, something you may not want if you hold a steady job or need to stay alert throughout the afternoon.[72] Those age forty and older, in particular, have been found to make more mistakes and feel sleepier after eating a high-carbohydrate lunch than after a high-protein lunch.[73] Italy, a land known for its laid back afternoons and siestas, feasts on pasta and bread at midday, a repast likely to stimulate large amounts of the calming yin chemical, serotonin. Japan, on the other hand, a country better known for their afternoon focus on work, is more likely to feature relatively more fish, a yang protein food, for lunch.

Non-starchy vegetables, such as broccoli, spinach, green beans, and zucchini, help keep our energy alive. The digestible carbohydrate content of these vegetables is relatively low and their levels of brain-stimulating nutrients and Qi-moving fiber are high. We know that cooked vegetables, which are rich in fiber and low in sugars, are relatively easy to digest, producing a smooth flow of Qi that we experience as good energy and the desire and fortitude to carry out our goals and dreams.

For afternoon energy, alertness, and productivity, the ideal midday meal choice should focus on meat, poultry, fish, or eggs—all energizing, yang foods. Vegetarians can choose from tofu, beans, peas, or lentils. Although less yang than animal products, legume choices are more energizing than starch-rich pastas or bread. Protein-rich foods, especially animal proteins, stimulate catecholamines, which are alertness brain chemicals that bolster energy, even when the body tends to cycle into its more relaxed state. Because morning is a time we naturally tend to be alert and more energized, having carbohydrates with protein (rice or toast with eggs, for example) provides balance for our most productive time.

Your evening meal can be chosen based on your post-dinner plans. If you're heading out for a PTA meeting or a movie after dinner, choose energizing protein foods so your brain catecholamines will keep you alert for your nighttime activities. If you want to relax after dinner, choose a serotonin-producing noodle- or rice-based meal with, of course, lots of vegetables.

SOURCES OF CARBOHYDRATE FOODS

All complex-carbohydrate foods nourish the spleen function, or digestion. They are particularly important foods for those who are frail and thin. Grains tend to benefit the elderly, children, and athletes most. In excess, however, grains can overburden the spleen, causing signs of indigestion, including gas and bloating. Below is a description of various carbohydrate-rich foods with explanations of both Chinese energetic patterns and Western nutritional properties.

Amaranth

Amaranth is a tiny, seedlike grain that cooks up into a delicious hot breakfast cereal or rice replacement. This highly nutritious protein- and calcium-rich grain was a sacred food of the Aztecs, cultivated about 7,000 years ago in Mexico. It is enjoyed in parts of Latin America and Africa for culinary, medicinal, magic, and religious purposes. A plant providing both a nutrient-dense edible seed-grain and a leaf, amaranth is particularly helpful in preventing malnutrition in impoverished parts of the world. In Asia, amaranth is grown on rugged hillsides scattered through the countryside.

With 18 percent of its calories from protein, amaranth is one of the most protein-rich grains known. Because of its lower carbohydrate content, amaranth is easier for most people to digest than wheat products. The calcium content of amaranth rivals that of milk. In its whole seed form, amaranth cooks in twenty to twenty-five minutes in water or broth (use two parts liquid to one part grain). It is also available in cold cereal flakes and as a type of flour. From a TCM perspective, amaranth is cooling. Its slight bitter flavor renders it drying and thus good for signs of dampness, yet it also possesses the properties to restore moisture to a pattern of dryness, making it a perfect food for someone with signs of both dampness and dryness (dry skin and hair, bloated stomach).

Barley

Perhaps dating as far back as rice, barley grows almost anywhere, from arctic Tibetan highlands to the parched Sahara desert. It comes in different forms, depending on the degree to which it is refined. Whole or Scotch barley has an intact bran, the nutrient- and oil-rich center. It is dark, rich, and chewy. Whole barley, because it is the least processed, is the most balancing and nutritious form of this grain. When unroasted, it can be a mild laxative. Pan-roasting barley makes it a good remedy for diarrhea. Pearl barley has had all of its bran, nutrients, and fiber removed, leaving only a small, white, starchy kernel. It's a poor choice from a nutritional standpoint.

Barley is cooling and moistening, thus balancing for dry signs. It is said to calm heat signs and to increase our yin fluids while at the same time clearing the tissues of excess fluids, or dampness. When ground, it can be made into a cooling tea, helpful in reducing signs of heat and fatigue from hot weather. Roasted or toasted barley is particularly drying and is thought to reduce swelling and tumors. Barley tends to be more easily digested than other grains, particularly wheat.

Buckwheat

No relation to wheat, buckwheat is technically not even a grain but rather a fruit. The flavor of buckwheat is bold and hearty, sometimes overpowering to the taste buds of Americans. It originated in North Central Asia and is one of the oldest and most traditional foods of Russia, where it is better known as kasha. Buckwheat is made into soba noodles in Japanese cuisine and into pancakes in America.

Its Western nutritional profile is similar to other grains. It is rich in B vitamins and particularly high in calcium, iron, and other minerals. Its high rutin (a flavonoid) content stimulates circulation, warming the hands and feet and reducing tendencies toward varicose veins and hemorrhoids. From a TCM perspective, the warming property of buckwheat, just like that of meats, makes it good for building blood. From a Western standpoint, both buckwheat and meats are iron-rich, making them good for preventing and treating anemia. Buckwheat also inhibits melanin, the protective tanning element in the skin, making it a better food for darker-complected people who are living in cold climates and have little exposure to sunlight (it is the staple grain of dark-skinned Siberians).

According to Chinese medicine, buckwheat is warming and thought to be beneficial in strengthening the stomach and digestion, especially in cases of dysentery. Buckwheat is also strengthening to the kidneys. It should not be consumed by those with heat or wind signs.

Corn

Corn, or maize as it is known throughout the world, is the only common native grain in the Western Hemisphere. Fossil pollen dates maize back 80,000 years. Like other grains, in appropriate amounts, corn is helpful to digestion, the heart, and the kidneys. It is slightly cooling and drying and thus balancing for those with patterns of heat and dampness. It makes a good replacement for breads and pasta in those with such patterns. As a cooling vegetable or grain, it also provides a pleasant balance to hot summer afternoons.

I vividly remember summertime and picking ears of sweet corn fresh from my garden, pulling the silky covering from the yellow ear to taste the unmatched sweetness of sun-warmed, right-off-the-plant corn. The sugar in corn almost immediately begins to change to starch when harvested, making it more a grain and less a vegetable the longer you wait for dinner. The deeper yellow and blue-colored varieties offer more nutrients than do the white kernels. Yellow corn contains more carotenoids than white. Blue corn contains 50 percent more iron, 21 percent more protein, and twice the manganese and potassium of yellow or white corn. All corn, however, is low in niacin and therefore a poor choice as a staple grain. Regular corn consumption should be supplemented with a diet rich in other whole grains, fish, and meats, all niacin-rich foods. Corn can be enjoyed fresh on the cob or as popcorn, polenta, grits, or tortillas.

Kamut

Kamut, another form of wheat, was grown in Egypt more than 5,000 years ago; it was later replaced with wheat products more similar to those we eat today. The story goes that a few kernels of kamut were recovered from an excavated tomb in Egypt in 1950, then planted by a farmer in Montana. His growing efforts have brought us the kamut flour, breads, and other products available as wheat alternatives today.

Kamut flour has similar baking properties to whole wheat. From a TCM perspective, this wheat-relative is also moistening but not quite as damp-producing as wheat. Unlike wheat, which is cooling, kamut is warming. This ancient grain is also richer in protein and unsaturated fats. Kamut also seems to cause fewer of the allergic symptoms associated with wheat. Tests show roughly two thirds those with wheat allergy have reduced or no allergic symptoms with kamut.[74]

Millet

Millet is a delicious, cooling, bright yellow, seed-like grain that makes an ideal hot breakfast cereal or replacement for rice. A staple of Asia, Africa, and India, millet originated in Eastern Asia and was an important food for northern China until the Tang Dynasty (A.D. 618–907).

Millet is richer in protein, B vitamins, magnesium, and several other minerals than are most grains, including oatmeal. According to TCM, it enhances digestion, as well as the kidneys' ability to provide the body with moist, cooling yin fluids. Thus it benefits patterns of dryness and heat. I particularly like millet on hot summer mornings—even though I eat it cooked and warm, its deep effect is to keep me cool and calm.

Millet has diuretic properties, yet it is also moistening to a pattern of dryness. It has anti-fungal properties, making it one of the few acceptable carbohydrate foods for those with Candida albicans (yeast) overgrowth. It is also therapeutic for morning sickness, and when roasted, beneficial for diarrhea.

Potatoes

Potatoes replace grains for many Americans and in some other cultures. Unlike grains, potatoes are extremely rich in vitamin C while being low in protein and B vitamins. They are neutral-to-cooling and moist—thus they are beneficial to those with patterns of heat and dryness. Like grains, potatoes nourish the spleen, or digestion, and thus our Qi energy. They are lubricating, supplying us with yin fluids. Potatoes are often easier to digest than many grains and so are often better tolerated by those with digestive problems such as bloating, gas, and indigestion.

Quinoa

The first time I experienced quinoa, I was visiting Peru. There, this delicate grain is incorporated into everything from soups to bread. A cousin to amaranth, quinoa is also from South America, dating back at least 8,000 years. Growing fast in popularity in this country as a culinary novelty, quinoa (pronounced KEEN-wa), is a highly nutritious, fine-grained seed (not part of the grass family of wheat and rice) that crackles something like tapioca pearls between your teeth when eaten boiled in its unprocessed state. Quinoa features a nutty, only slightly sweet flavor, with a barely detectable piquant aftertaste.

Quinoa is probably the most nutritious grain from a Western standpoint. Its protein content is an amazing 20 percent of its calories, roughly the same value as a cheeseburger. The World Health Organization states quinoa is equal or superior to milk as a protein source. It is also rich in B vitamins, iron, zinc, potassium, calcium, and vitamin E. Quinoa makes an excellent winter grain when cooked and served with poultry or lamb and vegetables.

From a Chinese medicine standpoint, quinoa is warming and strengthening, thus beneficial to someone with a cold pattern. It is particularly warming to the kidneys, making it an excellent food for vegetarians, the elderly, or anyone who feels cold, weak, or lacking in sexual energy. Additionally, its high essential-fat content gives quinoa a yin-building quality that makes it an excellent grain for someone with yin deficiency, or dryness. The high protein content of quinoa also supports the blood-sugar imbalances often present with dryness.

Rice

Rice is the staple grain for more than half the earth's population. In China, the word for rice is the same as that for food. Rice was probably the first grain, gathered by prehistoric people Southern Asia. It was thought to originate in India, spreading east to China and Indonesia. It first arrived in America in the late 1600s. Today, rice can be found from Asia to Italy, from Greece to Spain, including thousands of varieties—from Chinese black rice to Bhutanese red rice, from Bagladeshi Kalijira rice to Texas jasmine rice.

Rice is one of the most balanced of all foods. Although subtle differences among varieties do exist, most forms of rice are neither drying nor damp-producing, neither warming nor cooling. The few exceptions are wild and basmati rice, which tend to be slightly more drying than other types, and sweet rice, which has slight damp-forming properties. Thus most rice can be used in any pattern of imbalance. Rice makes an excellent replacement for wheat products for those with problems of dampness, including excess weight, sinus congestion, and digestive bloating and mucous. Rice strengthens the spleen, or digestion, and is often the only grain tolerated by those with certain digestive problems, including celiac sprue, irritable bowel syndrome, and Crohn's disease.

Most of the world eats polished, white rice. Naomi Duguid, who co-authored *Seductions of Rice* says, "We were '70s brown-rice eaters, but now you would call us rice eaters in a serious way, and rice eaters eat white rice."[75] There's great controversy in American nutrition circles over whether it's best to eat brown or white rice. From a Western perspective, white rice is a weak food. It's low in protein, fiber, and B-vitamins, nutrients we generally find in grains. No one would dispute that brown rice has more vitamins and minerals, as well as more fiber, than white rice, but the pertinent issue here is digestion. Those against eating brown rice complain it's too hard to digest. It needs to be chewed very thoroughly, something foreign to most Americans, who have problems with indigestion and dampness when eating brown rice. Interestingly, brown rice isn't consumed in Asia; white rice is the rice of choice throughout the Pacific Rim.

For those of my clients who take out too little time for meals and eating, I suggest white rice. For those with few digestive complaints, who lead a more relaxed lifestyle and who take time to savor, chew, and enjoy well-prepared meals, I encourage their use of brown rice. As for myself, I eat white rice on rushed days or when there is a veritable feast of choices before me, such as at a banquet or party. I prepare brown rice when I can relax in the quiet of my kitchen and enjoy it with a simple, stir-fried vegetable dish.

Spelt

Spelt originated in Southeast Asia and was brought to the Middle East over 9,000 years ago. Saint Hildegard of Bingen, a twelfth-century mystic, claimed spelt could heal people who were so sick they could not eat. She found spelt to be the grain best tolerated by the body. It is actually used today to treat digestive problems, nerve disorders, and even cancer in the Hildegard Practice Clinic in Germany.

This ancient form of wheat is generally easier to digest than wheat itself. For those with wheat allergies and symptoms such as irritable bowel syndrome, gas, bloating, or indigestion, spelt offers an alternative, in the form of bread or pasta, that's sometimes even healing. As you might expect, instead of being cooling like wheat, spelt is warming and strengthening to the spleen (digestion). It is also moistening and helps a pattern of dryness. You can find spelt breads, pasta, cereals, and flours.

Wheat

The most widely consumed grain in the United States is without doubt wheat. It is everywhere—in breads, cereals, cookies, crackers, and baked goods. Indeed, the most widely distributed grain in the world is wheat, with over 30,000 varieties. It is grown in every country and has origins in Jericho over 10,000 years ago with primitive wheat forms: einkorn and emmer. The European colonists first brought wheat to America; it was in a form not easily grown in the area so was modified.

In 1880, Pillsbury figured out how to strip whole wheat of its nutrient-rich germ, fiber, essential fatty acids, vitamins, and minerals, leaving a white, starchy, empty-calorie powder known as flour. Today, several types of wheat are commonly available: hard (usually made into breads), soft (usually made into white-flour pastries and baked goods), durum (good for pasta), and semolina (also used for pasta).

From our morning toast to our midday sandwiches and evening spaghetti with garlic sourdough, we live on wheat. Whether it's the refined white flour that goes into our soft white bread sandwiches or the whole sprouted wheat that goes into our dense, grainy brown loaves, we are overeating it. Many Western health authorities consider wheat to be the main culprit in food allergies, along with digestive problems (bloating), fluid retention, sinus congestion, and obesity.

From a TCM perspective, wheat is cooling and damp. Those qualities make noodles and bread potentially good foods for someone frail and underweight. However, these same qualities when taken in at virtually every meal can lead to weight gain—excess fat is dampness. Wheat can cause mucous to accumulate in the sinuses and digestive tract, with bloating and indigestion often occurring in the abdomen.

From a Western perspective, the same food eaten day after day may, in some, contribute to allergies. It makes sense that we are designed to flourish on seasonally available foods, such as tomatoes and melons in summer, apples and squash in fall, and meats and root vegetables in winter. Repeatedly eating the same food day after day not only reduces the variety of nutrients possible in our diets but may provoke an immune system response that leaves us with digestion or sinus problems. Ideally, we should give our systems a break from foods that we habitually eat.

Another problem with wheat is that it has been genetically altered over the years, making life easier for farmers and food processors, yet more difficult for our delicate digestive systems. With its essential fat-rich germ center, wheat is also very perishable. Processed, stored whole wheat is often rancid and contributes to a host of health problems associated with poor-quality fats.

The nutritional value of wheat is higher when it is consumed whole, fresh, and minimally processed. Sprouted or freshly ground wheat berries cooked in water or made into bread provide significantly more magnesium, manganese, iron, B vitamins, and fiber than do white-flour products.

Two ancient forms of wheat—kamut and spelt (both described above)—are becoming more readily available and recognized as more easily digestible and less allergy-promoting forms of this grain. They are made into breads, pasta, and other foods traditionally made with wheat.

Wild Rice

Wild rice, called "manomin" or "good berry" by the Chippewa and other Algonquin tribes, is not a true rice. Rather, it is the seed of an aquatic grass, the only wild grain commercially available in America, though most wild rice is commercially grown in California. Truly wild rice, which grows in the Great Lakes region, offers a wider range of dramatic flavors and aromas than the cultivated type. Wild rice is richer in protein, iron, B vitamins, and fiber than real rice and is particularly beneficial as a replacement to other grains for weight loss. This drying, cooling seed served as a staple to many Native American people, contributing to their tall, muscular physiques.

---

72. Wurtman, Judith, *Managing Your Mind and Mood Through Food*. Rawson Associates (1986): 70.
73. Ibid.
74. Ibid.
75. Duguid, Naomi, *Seductions of Rice*. New York: Artisan, 1998.

13

SUGARS:
SWEET NOTHINGS OR KILLERS?

I'm convinced that one of our worst dietary habits is our refined-sugar intake. Many people would find relief from their mood swings, health problems, and excess weight if they could just get rid of the sweets. But Americans love their sugar.

Sugar is hot and damp, according to TCM theory. Unlike grains and starchy vegetables, which tend to be neutral or even cooling, sugar is heating, a yang quality. Although initially, in some people, sugar has a calming and sedating, yin-like effect, sodas and other sweets can ultimately provoke agitation, aggression, and irritability. Western research shows that a high-sugar snack can trigger rebound low blood sugar, which stimulates the release of adrenaline, a hormone that may provoke aggressiveness and hostility, both hot, yang imbalances.

In the West, we recognize sugar as an empty-calorie food. We know that overuse of sugar can lead to tooth decay and obesity. It is also associated with hyperactivity, anxiety, behavioral problems, diabetes, heart disease, arthritis, eczema, PMS, cancer, acne, and digestive problems, to name a few conditions.[76] In TCM, sugar is associated with patterns of heat and of dampness, encompassing many of the very conditions linked with sugar intake from a Western perspective.

From a Chinese perspective, sugar's damp and heating nature can provoke anger, excess weight gain, yellow mucous, red skin rashes and acne, PMS symptoms, and indigestion with gas. And both Western and Chinese nutritionists link overuse of sugar to common symptoms such as obesity, candida or yeast infections, sinus congestion, abdominal bloating, herpes, canker sores, and pus-filled acne, all signs of dampness.

The damp, heating nature of sugar (from a TCM standpoint) and insulin-elevating property (from a Western perspective) implicate it in diabetes, breast cancer, high blood pressure, and heart disease, including elevated cholesterol and triglyceride levels, conditions associated with other heating foods such as fatty meats, fried foods, and saturated fat.

OUR INTAKE OF SUGAR

Americans eat around 139 pounds of sugar per capita each year, in the form of refined white sugar, brown sugar, raw sugar, high-fructose syrup, fructose, corn sweeteners, fruit juice, and syrups. That's two thirds of a cup of sugar per day. Soft drinks provide one quarter of this amount. Jelly beans, chocolates, cinnamon rolls, jam, ice cream, cookies, and other sweets provide the rest. Our sugar intake increased by twenty-five pounds from 1970 to 1996, roughly the same period obesity increased by thirty percent.[77]

Americans drank twice as many soft drinks in 1997 as in 1973 and 43 percent more than in 1985. The fast-food industry is propelling us in the direction of increasing sugar consumption. Interestingly, and sadly, in 1997 Coca-Cola spent $277 million on advertising, whereas the National Cancer Institute spent just $1 million on the "Five a Day Program," encouraging us to eat more vegetables and fruits.

POPULAR HIGH-SUGAR FOODS	TEASPOONS OF SUGAR
3 Musketeers, 2.1 oz.	10
Au Bon Pain blueberry muffin	9
Ben & Jerry's Devil's FoodChocolate Sorbet, 1 cup	16.5

POPULAR HIGH-SUGAR FOODS	**TEASPOONS OF SUGAR**
Cinnabon	12.25
Coca-Cola, 12 oz.	10
Dairy Queen Chocolate Shake, medium	28.5
Entemann's Light Fudge Iced Chocolate Cake, 1/6th	8.25
Frosted Flakes, 1 cup	4.30
Häagen Däzs Chocolate-Chocolate Chip Ice Cream, 1 cup	12
Junior Mints, 1.6 oz. box	9.25
M&M's, 1.7 oz.	7.75
McDonald's Hot Fudge Sundae	11.75
Mountain Dew, 8 oz.	12
Ocean Spray Cranapple, 8 oz.	7.25
Oreos, 3	3.25
SnackWell's Fat Free Devil's Food Cake, 2	3.5
Snapple Pink Lemonade, 8 oz.	6.75
Sunkist Orange Soda, 8 oz.	13
Twinkies, 2	7

Source: Nutrition Action, Volume 25, Number 9, November 1998

Ten Ways to Cut Sugar Cravings

Most people do consider sugar a healthful food. The problem is just how to stop yearning for those chocolates, jelly beans, and brownies. The following steps will actually reduce your desire for sweets by altering the chemistry of your blood and brain, including stabilizing blood sugar and stimulating serotonin and other brain chemicals that keep you content without a cookie. Many of these dietary principles are part of the Chinese way of life.

1. Have a non-sweet breakfast containing a protein-rich food. Choose a whole grain plus the appropriate protein source for your body: eggs, lox, smoked fish, lean poultry sausage, soy products, beans, nuts, or seeds.
2. Include adequate high-quality protein at lunch. Again, choose the protein-rich foods best for your body pattern: eggs, fish, poultry, lean beef or pork, nuts, seeds, or legumes.
3. Avoid excess raw fruits, raw vegetables, and juice. (Fruits and

especially juices are high in sugars, which can leave your blood sugar low, and create a desire for more sweets.) Raw fruits and vegetables are also energetically very cooling, a quality that can drive up your desire for foods that are warming, such as sugar.

4. Include cooked leafy greens daily, especially if chocolate cravings are a problem.

5. Drink green tea daily. It helps to maintain stable blood sugar levels thereby minimizing cravings for sugar.

6. Avoid artificial sweeteners. Your body may respond as if they are actually real sugars.

7. Bite the bullet and reduce or eliminate refined sugars (sucrose, fructose, fruit juice, honey, and syrups).

8. Get adequate full-spectrum lighting. Natural light is essential for the brain to produce serotonin, the calming brain chemical that prevents sugar cravings. Take a twenty-minute walk outdoors in the early morning, sit near a bright window, or use full-spectrum lighting in your workspace.

9. Include an essential-fat source such as flax, pumpkin, or hemp seed oils, fish oils, or DHA and EPA oils.

10. Try supplements of magnesium (350–500 mg.) and chromium (200–500 mcg.), minerals that stabilize blood sugar, or the herbs gymnema sylvestre or fennel leaf, or licorice root. (Licorice root tastes sweet plus it stimulates the adrenals, which can boost energy in someone with weak adrenals. In large amounts licorice may raise blood pressure, however and should be used with caution.)

SUGAR AND HEART DISEASE

According to William B. Grant, PhD, simple sugar is the primary diet-related risk factor in heart disease. He explains that sugars are incorporated into triglycerides, which then form very low-density lipoproteins (VLDLs), the most hazardous form of cholesterol. One study revealed that by removing white sugar from the diet, serum-cholesterol levels could drop from 230 to 190 mg/dl in a month, and that if sugars were added back into the diet, cholesterol levels would again rise.[78] Grant contends that dietary fat's implication in heart-disease risk is based on flawed research.[79]

Thus, contrary to popular opinion, excess sugar consumption may contribute more to heart disease than does fat consumption.[80] Indeed, Harvard researchers found that the most important factor for determining heart-disease risk is probably not high cholesterol levels, which we associate with overeating saturated fats, but rather obesity, high blood pressure, and high triglyceride levels, all of which reflect insulin levels and sugar intake.[81] The TCM perspective on sugar corroborates these Western conclusions.

SUGAR AND EXCESSIVE INSULIN RELEASE

Many of the problems associated with sugar stem from its tendency to overstimulate insulin, a growth and fat-storage hormone and thus a potential contributor to dampness when produced in excess. When you are healthy, the pancreas (the Western organ) releases insulin whenever you eat. Insulin sweeps sugars, fats, and proteins from the blood, packing them into cells, where they are burned for energy or stored for later use. Adequate levels of this hormone are critical to keeping our blood-sugar levels from getting too high, as is the case with diabetes. Overproduction of insulin can drive our blood sugar levels too low, as in the situation of hypoglycemia.

A condition called insulin resistance occurs when the cells of the liver, fat, and muscle fail to respond to normal levels of insulin, thus keeping sugars and other nutrients from entering cells, the body's energy-producing metabolic chambers. Higher and higher levels of insulin need to be released by the pancreas to do the same job. We can develop insulin resistance from too much stress, getting fat, overeating poor-quality fats, and not getting enough essential fats, as well as from overeating calories in general or sugar in particular.

Too much insulin comes with a number of health problems. The greater the insulin level, the higher the likelihood of obesity, high blood pressure, breast cancer, heart disease,[82] diabetes, and cancer, all damp conditions.[83] Excess insulin causes your body to make more of the inflammatory prostaglandin, arachidonic acid (covered in detail in chapter eleven), which can lead to worsening arthritis pain, headaches, PMS symptoms, and irritable bowel flare ups. A high sugar intake and resulting high insulin levels are also associated with higher breast cancer risk. Insulin may work as a growth factor along with estrogen in promoting breast tumors.[84] Tumors, according to TCM, are damp masses, areas where our Qi gets stuck and dampness is allowed to accumulate. The damp nature of foods made with sugar may contribute to areas of tumor growth. High insulin levels also reduce blood-sugar levels to energy-depleting lows, leaving us lethargic and often wanting more sugar.

When blood sugar and insulin levels remain too high for an extended period, insulin resistance worsens, making weight loss more and more difficult, which further contributes to high blood pressure and triglyceride levels, and risk of heart disease. According to Stanford University professor Gerald Reaven, 25 percent of the population is insulin resistant, including most of those with diabetes and half those with high blood pressure.

SUGAR AND OBESITY

In addition to its role in the above-mentioned health problems, insulin is a fat-storage hormone. Higher than normal levels of insulin increase a tendency to obesity. Being overly fat further contributes to insulin resistance, making weight loss increasingly difficult. A high level of insulin contributes to making us fat in two ways: As a hormone that encourages the storage of nutrients, insulin is involved in creating dampness in the form of body fat. From the Western standpoint, it increases lipoprotein lipase, an enzyme that stores fat. It also inactivates hormone-sensitive lipase, an enzyme that breaks down stored fat. In an obese person, insulin is elevated all the time, creating a tenacious pattern of weight gain with difficulty losing it.[85]

HOW SUGAR AFFECTS MOOD AND PERFORMANCE

According to the Chinese concept of sugar leading to dampness, when the mist of dampness rises, it creates a feeling of mental fogginess, including memory loss. Sugar, from our Western viewpoint, can lead to a feeling of mental cloudiness, including forgetfulness. Some researchers implicate an allergic reaction to sugar and its mind-impairing potential. Because sugary foods are devoid of nutrients, sweets require nutrients from other foods for their assimilation, in particular increasing our need for B vitamins, nutrients involved in production of brain chemicals that facilitate mental clarity, learning, and stable moods.

Sugar also stimulates cortisol and adrenaline, two stress hormones associated with anxiety and aggression. Cortisol is also thought to interfere with loss of short- and long-term memory.

From a TCM perspective, the damp nature of sugar can leave us with damp signs such as depression, excess weight, and overproduction of estrogen, our most yin hormone. Depression, a yin mental state, relative to a sunny outlook, may result from a diet too rich in yin, or damp foods. Larry Christensen, Chairman of the Department of Psychiatry at the University of Alabama, found depressed patients who cut out sugar and caffeine reported their energy levels went up within one week. Depression also lifted.

The feeling of imbalance created by eating sugary food leads many, particularly women, to reach for more and more sugar to ease the unpleasant effects of eating it in the first place. It may come as little surprise that the foods women most crave are those with the most sugar, such as chocolate, cookies, and ice cream. Sugar and fat-rich foods stimulate the release of endorphins, brain chemicals related to morphine that leave a pleasant, relaxing feeling.

HIGH GLYCEMIC-INDEX FOODS

Not only can overeating sugar, specifically, lead to insulin resistance, but also overeating in general, as well as alcohol overuse and eating bad fats, drives up blood-sugar and thus insulin levels, leading to greater risk of disease. Thus, overindulging in French fries, donuts, candy, cookies, soft drinks, and other fatty and sugar-rich foods tends to lead to health problems. These foods have a higher *glycemic index*. As discussed in the introduction, it is generally accepted that the more high glycemic-index foods consumed, the greater the rise in insulin levels and the higher the likelihood of obesity, high blood pressure, heart disease, diabetes, and even cancer, all damp conditions.[86] High glycemic index foods are most often refined sweets such as jelly beans, colas, ice cream, cakes, and frozen yogurt, yet they can also be complex carbohydrates, such as bread and crackers, and even "bad" fats.

Foods with the highest glycemic index and thus the greatest threat to health include white bread, pretzels, instant rice, rice cakes, bagels, flaked cereals, potatoes, and French fries. The high glycemic index of these foods causes glucose, and thus insulin, to be released in greater quantities than it is by other foods. Breads, noodles, and other sources of wheat may elevate insulin levels more readily than do other carbohydrate foods with similar nutritional properties.[87]

Relatively recent research reveals that certain fatty foods, in particular those rich in saturated and hydrogenated fats, can have a higher glycemic index than some carbohydrate foods.[88] Margarine, vegetable shortening, and other sources of hydrogenated fats, as well as beef and pork fat, dairy fat, and other sources of saturated fats, seem particularly able to stimulate insulin levels.

High levels of these fats in the blood may contribute to the escalation of the harmful VLDL cholesterol, triglycerides, and cholesterol levels associated with increased risk of heart disease.[89] The combination of fat and sugar in bakery products seems to promote a particularly high glycemic index.[90] From the TCM perspective, both sweets and saturated fat-rich foods are damp.

Not only are they likely to produce high glucose and insulin levels, they also produce a detrimental byproduct as a result of the baking process. When sugar is baked along with milk and flour, a reaction called browning, or the Maillard reaction, occurs, in which the chemical modification of proteins by sugars leaves them nutritionally unavailable and potentially able to block digestive enzymes.[91] Physicians called the browning reaction glycosylation, and research associates it in the body with diseases of aging, including aged skin, arteries, and other tissues, which means greater risk for heart disease, cancer, and dementia. In addition, the absorption of these new, fragmented proteins may trigger allergic reactions, including bloating, water retention, and sinus congestion—all signs of dampness in TCM. From the TCM perspective, baked products such as cookies, cakes, and muffins are especially a problem for those with signs of dampness. Indeed, any interference with digestion can lead to damp signs.

The correlation between glycemic index and dampness in susceptible individuals becomes even more closely tied in light of observations by Jeffery Bland, PhD, Nutrition Researcher and founder of HealthComm, International. According to his research, certain foods can produce very high levels of insulin in some people and not in others. From the standpoint of TCM, someone with a predisposition to dampness will see their weight climb and perhaps their sinuses congest more readily than someone with a pattern of dryness, reinforcing the Western idea of biochemical individuality.

Low glycemic index foods include beans, lentils, tofu, poultry, fish, eggs, nuts, seeds, and unprocessed whole grains. In general, whole grains have a lower glycemic index than their processed versions; whole-wheat bread causes a slower release of sugar into the bloodstream than does white bread. Studies show that the more whole grains people eat, the better able they are to lower their fasting insulin levels, their rate of obesity, and their tendency toward an apple shape—the body shape most associated with heart disease.[92]

---

76. Gittleman, Ann Louise, MS, CNS, *Get The Sugar Out*. New York: Crown, 1996, pp. xxvi, xxvii

77. Winitz, Seedman, DA, "Studies in Metabolic Nutrition Employing Chemically Defined Diets," *Am Jr of Clin Nutr,* 23 (1970): 525–43.

78. Winitz, Seedman, DA, "Studis in Metabolic Nutrition Employing Chemically Defined Diets," *Am Jr of Clin Nutr,* 23 (1970): 525–43.

79,80. Grant, William "The Role of Sugars in Ischemic Heart Disease," *The Townsend Letter for Doctors and Patients* (February/March 1999): 80.

81,82. *Circulation* 98 (August 4, 1998): 398–404.

83,84. Yam, D., "Insulin-Cancer Relationship: Possible Dietary Implication," *Medical Hypothesis* 38 (1992): 111–17.

85. Steward, Bethea, and Balart Andrews, *Sugar Busters*. New York: Ballantine Books (1998) 54 55.

86,87. Yam, D., "Insulin-Cancer Relationship: Possible Dietary Implication," *Medical Hypothesis* 38 (1992): 111–17.

88,89. Simopoulos, Artemis, P., "s Insulin Resistance Influenced by Dietary Linoleic Acid and Trans Fatty Acids," *Free Radical Biology and Medicine* 17(4) (1994): 367–72.

90,91. Holt, Suzanne, "An Insulin Index of Foods," *American Journal of Clinical Nutrition* 66 (1997): 1264–76.

92. Jancin, Bruce, "Whole Grain May Reduce Obesity, Hyperinsulinemia," *Family Practice News* (May 15, 1998): 8.

14

VEGETABLES AND FRUITS
FOR BALANCE

※

People in other countries eat more vegetables than we do. The plant-based diet of China is the key to its protection against our Western diseases, according to T. Collin Campbell, the Cornell researcher who has been studying the Chinese and their diet since 1983. A generous intake of vegetables, fruits, grains, and soy products is credited with keeping the cholesterol levels among mainland Chinese to a level roughly half ours, while holding obesity, heart disease, and cancer rates to fractions of ours in the United States.

When I was in China, I saw vegetables prepared and served at every meal. In fact, they made up the bulk of each meal. We had bok choy, bamboo shoots, and bean sprouts at breakfast. Dinner and lunch were feasts of Chinese broccoli, pea pods, green beans, carrots, squashes, eggplant, cabbage, and various other root and green leafy vegetables. Vegetables were stir fried, stewed, and simmered. They were made into soups, pickled salads, and noodles dishes. Rice and small amounts of animal foods accompanied this colorful plethora of vegetables.

One day while I was in Beijing, I discovered a rich and satisfying vegetable snack when a vendor pushing a large cooking barrel sold me a freshly roasted sweet potato tucked into a folded paper cone. The potato's sweet warm flesh was easily squeezed from its skin, making it a practical, nutritious, and flavorful snack.

FOODS FOR LONG LIFE AND HAPPINESS

Perhaps the only area in nutrition in which there's no controversy is the recommendation to eat vegetables and fruits—and lots of them, preferably in season. The reasons for this advice are many. Vegetables and fruits are excellent sources of fiber, which provides satiety, speeds calories through the body, helps keep intestines clean and free of toxins, reduces absorption of cholesterol and hormones, and protects against diverticulitis, polyps, and certain types of cancer.

The best choice for vegetables and fruits is organic. Possible benefits include less pesticide residues needing to be processed by your liver, higher concentrations of nutrients, and better flavor. Unfortunately there isn't much focus on the importance of organic foods in Chinese medicine, perhaps because use of pesticides, antibiotics and other chemical additives is relatively recent. Also, the focus of Chinese medicine is really the art of balancing the energetic properties of foods. The health benefits of vegetables and fruits, even if laced with pesticides, far outweigh the risks of a diet low in these foods. In fact, animal fat, including milk fat, accumulates more pesticides than vegetables do.

That said, there is an alarming association between the chemicals used in our foods and the incidence of cancers, infertility, and other related health problems. There is an estimated 800,000 cases of acute intoxication, including 3,000 deaths from pesticides worldwide each year.[93] The EPA is so concerned, they are planning a study of approximately 87,000 chemicals that are believed to upset the body's hormone balance. Some animal and human studies suggest pesticides may be hazardous to the developing brain at levels of exposure far below those required to cause symptoms. Pesticides are designed to be toxins, to kill their target organism, be it an insect, plant or animal.

Because many pesticides mimic hormones, they are suspected of increasing risk of prostate cancer in men[94] and breast cancer in women. In one recent study, women in the upper three quartiles of hexachlorobenzene, a pesticide, were at twice the risk of breast cancer as those in the lowest quartile.[95]

Fruits and vegetables particularly prone to accumulating large pesticide residues include peaches, pears, green beans, spinach, apples, celery, strawberries, winter squash, and peppers. To reduce your pesticide exposure, wash all fruits and vegetables in soapy water, peel fruits that can be peeled, and buy organic whenever possible.

Fruits and vegetables are significant contributors of anti-aging, anti-cancer, heart-protective nutrients. Antioxidants, for instance, including vitamins C and E, beta-carotene, some of the B vitamins, the mineral selenium, and other plant chemicals, protect our cells from damage by daily reactions involving oxygen. Nutrients and oxygen are processed continuously by the cells of our blood, heart, liver, brain, and other tissues, resulting in formation of toxic byproducts, including chemicals called free radicals. These reactive chemicals are associated with plaque build-up on artery walls and thus heart disease, cancer, cataracts, and the aging process itself. Studies show foods rich in antioxidant nutrients, including fruits and vegetables, are highly protective against a variety of cancers, atherosclerosis, heart disease, cataracts, arthritis, dementia, and inflammation—conditions associated with the damage brought on by oxidation and the aging process.

Potassium, a mineral found abundantly in vegetables, has recently been found to be highly protective against high blood pressure and stroke. Low potassium intake may play a role in the high blood pressure that affects forty-three million Americans. A Harvard School of Public Health Study with 44,000 men over eight years found those who ate nine servings of potassium-rich vegetables and fruits per day had one third fewer strokes than those who ate just four servings or fewer per day.[96] We need 3,500 milligrams of potassium per day to reduce risk of disease. To get that much, we should have at least four to six cups of potassium-rich vegetables, fruits, or legumes each day. Particularly good sources are lima beans, potatoes, spinach, avocado, and bananas.

Broccoli family vegetables, such as kale, broccoli, broccoli rabe, and mustard greens, can be found in many Chinese dishes. Along with antioxidants and carotenoids, these vegetables contain sulforaphane, a chemical that fights cancer. Sulforaphane is believed to energize an enzyme that breaks down cancer-causing substances, a remarkably close description of how Qi might be described in dissolving damp masses (including tumors), according to Chinese medical thought.

RAW VEGETABLES AND FRUITS

Many people believe there's nothing more healthful than a salad or a piece of fruit. For some people, these can be ideal food choices for balance. Yet for others, raw vegetables and raw fruits contribute to indigestion, abdominal bloating and gas, cravings, fluid retention, weight gain, fatigue, and even illness.

Keep in mind that eating large salads and salad-based meals is unique to America, a country with one of the highest obesity rates and widespread digestive problems. Entrées of mixed raw greens, chef's salads, seafood salads, Caesar salads, and other salad meals are not part of traditional European fare and are virtually unheard of in most of Asia. Other cultures prefer warm, cooked foods at mealtime, perhaps accompanied by a small salad or pickled vegetable.

From a TCM perspective, too many salads and other raw foods are hard on digestion, weakening spleen Qi, causing dampness, and leading to a host of digestive problems, weight gain, and low energy. Unlike cooked vegetables, raw fruit and salads are particularly cooling and should be minimized by those with a cold or a damp pattern and especially by anyone with a combination of cold and dampness. Those with a pattern of heat, on the other hand, often feel better when they switch to lighter fare of salads and fruits. The cooling quality of raw produce balances the heat resulting from years of eating fatty meats, fried and spicy foods, cheese, and alcohol.

Caution is advised in feasting on salads and raw fruits for those with patterns of cold, dampness, or dryness. Too many cold, raw foods can diminish the warming, yang energy we need for digestion. Fruits, and in particular, fruit juices, are particularly damp for the digestion and may, when eaten to excess, contribute to abdominal bloating, fluid retention, and weight gain. The sugars in fruits tend to draw fluid into the digestive tract. In those with a pattern of dryness, the sugars in fruit may further contribute to low blood sugar and therefore sugar cravings and energy fluctuations.

Cooked fruits and vegetables are more easily assimilated and deliver more nutrients than their raw versions. From a Chinese perspective, this makes them beneficial to spleen Qi and thus our metabolism, our ability to generate energy and to burn fat. Salads, when they begin to weaken spleen Qi, are really slowing digestion and potentially contributing excess weight gain.

Eating cooked foods flies in the face of recommendations by raw-food enthusiasts who say it's harmful to cook vegetables because heat destroys essential nutrients. While cooking foods does destroy some nutrients, light cooking leaves most nutrients intact and, even more important, more easily absorbed. Those nutrients remaining after cooking are often much better assimilated than are the nutrients in raw foods, leaving body tissues with better access to their healing properties.

Lycopene, for instance, a plant pigment found in tomatoes, is particularly beneficial to men in reducing risk of prostate cancer. Absorption of lycopene through the digestive system can be increased with cooked sources such as tomato sause. Cooking allows for the release of this nutrient from where it is found tightly bound to fiber and protein in vegetables.

In a study at the University of California, Berkeley, researchers compared the absorption of vitamin C from raw versus cooked broccoli. It was found that those who ate their broccoli lightly cooked saw blood levels of vitamin C go up 20 percent higher than those who ate the vegetable raw. Cooking apparently softens the cell wall of vegetables, allowing more nutrients into the blood.

Even Western research suggests that it may even be unhealthy, in some cases, to eat certain plant foods raw. Andrew Weil, MD, author of several books on nutrition and health, including 8 *Weeks to Optimal Health*, says, "It's important to eat lots of fruits and vegetables, but I don't think it is healthy to eat all raw foods. The best diet is a varied diet, and this goes for methods of preparation as well. Cooking renders foods more digestible; it also breaks down natural toxins that are in some vegetables and seeds." He goes on to say, "If you're not feeling well, raw vegetables can make things worse. They are especially hard on an irritated colon."[97]

In his web site, Dr. Weil points out that toxins in a number of foods are destroyed by cooking. Alfalfa sprouts contain a toxin called canavanine. Celery, especially any brownish or bruised area, harbors toxins that may sensitize us to sunlight and damage our immune systems. Raw spinach, chard, and beet greens contain higher amounts oxalic acid, which robs your body of calcium and iron, than cooked versions of those greens do. Cultivated white mushrooms contain several carcinogens. Members of the cabbage family also contain toxins, including thyroid-inhibiting compounds. "In general," says Dr. Weil, "these natural toxins are destroyed by cooking, especially cooking in water."

Science may have unveiled a mechanism by which salads interfere with weight loss. In a presentation given to other physicians, Richard Kunin, MD, a nutrition-oriented medical doctor and author in San Francisco, explains that a wax-like form of fat found on the leaves of raw lettuce, spinach, and other leaves can accumulate in the blood and cause problems with energy levels and weight loss. When excess salads are eaten, this waxy substance builds up and prevents fat from being burned effectively. This leaf wax works as a roadblock of sorts, preventing fat from getting to the body's cellular combustion chamber, or mitochondria, where it is burned for energy. Dr. Kunin reports that patients who eat lots of salads develop a pattern of low energy, difficulty losing weight, and cravings for sweets. When fat isn't burned, it shows up on your hips, thighs, and belly; your energy level dives; and you feel like eating, even if you aren't actually in need of food.

Overeating fruits, including meals of fruit salad or a fruit smoothie, can be a particular problem, especially if you're plagued by sugar cravings. Not only are such fruit-rich feasts very cooling to digestion, they are rich in sugars that can send your blood sugar, energy, and mood on a roller coaster ride. Consuming too many fruits and juices in some cases can stimulate excess insulin, which drives down blood sugar and thus energy levels, leaving the urge for more sweets as a pick-me-up.

The body craves balance. According to Chinese wisdom, when we eat too many cooling foods, the body responds by urging us to reach for the opposite—warming foods. Refined sugars found in cookies, cake, candy, and muffins are warming. The cooling qualities of too many raw fruits, juices, and salads stimulate a desire for a balance from the warming nature of such sweets.

BALANCE AND POWER WITH LEAFY GREENS

One of the most important healing foods is the broad category of dark leafy greens: bok choy, broccoli, spinach, kale, and mustard greens, as well as the green food concentrates: blue-green algae, chlorella, spirulina, and various young grasses. I've often thought leafy green vegetables should be a food group in and of themselves, just like dairy products or breads. All mammals, when diseased, switch to a diet of grass and other tender greens to soothe digestive ailments or rid their bodies of toxins.

Leafy green vegetables such as broccoli and spinach are packed with some of the most powerful nutrients we know of. They are among the best sources of antioxidants, including beta-carotene and vitamin E. Greens are rich in the nutrients most lacking in the Western diet, including magnesium, calcium, folic acid, fiber, and essential fats. These nutrients have been found to be most important in preventing the top killers in Western cultures: cardiovascular disease, stroke, and cancer, as well as the diseases and tissue damage associated with aging. Other lifesaving nutrients particularly rich in greens include potassium, various phytochemicals, and fiber.

The Chinese include leafy greens daily in their diets. When I visited China, I saw at least one choice of leafy green vegetable at every meal, including breakfast. In fact, most cultures include some kind of cooked dark leafy green daily. In Italy, it's called *verdura*. In Holland the term *greonte* refers to the color green as well as to green vegetables, an important part of the diet there. A client of mine, who recently returned to the United States after living in Brazil for two years, told me almost every restaurant and household where she had lived routinely served a kale dish in which this leafy green is cut finely, then sautéed with garlic and olive oil. The Chinese would say leafy green vegetables are uplifting and energizing because they grow rapidly and outward toward the sun. According to TCM, fresh leafy greens stimulate life energy, or Qi. A Western explanation would be that greens contain chlorophyll. The dark green color of vegetables comes from chlorophyll, and at the center of the chlorophyll molecule is magnesium, the mineral that goes into forming ATP, the chemical form of energy in the body. According to Paul Pitchford in *Healing with Whole Foods*, chlorophyll benefits anemic conditions, reduces high blood pressure, strengthens the intestines, relieves nervousness, and works as a diuretic.

Greens are important for all patterns of imbalance. Despite their delicious taste, most leafy green vegetables are nevertheless considered "bitter" in flavor, making them cooling and drying. This makes greens an excellent choice for weight and fat loss as well as for eliminating excess fluids. Exceptions are spinach and Swiss chard, which are considered more "sweet" than bitter, and thus better choices for moistening a dry or yin-deficient pattern. Some greens are also slightly warming and thus best for those with signs of cold. Warming greens include asparagus, broccoli rabe, kale, and mustard greens. All green vegetables, and particularly green food concentrates, are considered therapeutic, calming and cooling to the liver, and thus beneficial for those with heat signs such as anger, impatience, frustration, PMS (with anger), and headaches.

Leafy green vegetables provide other important nutrients, including calcium, a nutrient associated mainly with dairy products. Dairy products are not part of the traditional diet in China, where osteoporosis rates are lower than in dairy-consuming Western countries. Many greens are richer in calcium than milk products are, plus they contain co-factors that help assimilate calcium and build bone, including vitamin K, a nutrient required by a bone-building protein. Without adequate vitamin K, risk of bone-weakening conditions such as osteoporosis may increase. One cup of boiled collard greens provides more calcium than a cup of 1-percent milk. Additionally, the high magnesium content and low protein content of collards renders them a more available and readily assimilated form of calcium than milk.

All greens are a good source of calcium; however, if you're looking to greens as your calcium source, don't rely on spinach, Swiss chard, and beet greens. These contain oxalic acid, a compound that may interfere with calcium assimilation, especially when eaten raw. Consider spinach, chard, and beet greens as a healthy food, rich in iron, magnesium, and B vitamins, to be enjoyed frequently but not as your main source of calcium nor your regular form of leafy greens. Better choices for bone building include kale, mustard greens, turnip greens, and broccoli.

Green vegetables are also rich in folic acid, a vitamin associated with protection from spinal defects, a variety of cancers, brain damage, and heart disease. Adequate folic acid enables the body to overcome a common genetic mutation leading to increased risk of both spinal defects and cardiovascular disease.[98] Although these appear to be very different conditions, they seem to develop by a similar mechanism, and folic acid prevents this process. Folic acid, in particular, prevents the build-up of homocysteine, a compound that when produced in the body at high levels is associated with heart attack, high blood pressure, and stroke.

The 1998 National Health and Nutrition Examination Survey Epidemiological Follow-up Study, with 3,059 adults, found that low levels of folic acid were associated with mortality from not just cardiovascular disease but from all causes.[99] We're not taking in enough of this invaluable nutrient to protect us from these major health problems. The Center for Disease Control reports from five to 33 percent of the U.S. population may not be taking in adequate folic acid.[100] Sixty-eight to 87 percent of females of child bearing age have folic acid intakes below the recommended intake of 400 micrograms per day.[101] The recommended amount of folic acid to prevent such health problems is 400 micrograms. Just one cup of cooked spinach provides 262 micrograms of folic acid, and ten spears of asparagus provides 240 micrograms, each over half the recommended levels.

To get the full benefit of leafy green vegetables, they need to be dark and they need to be cooked. Iceberg salads don't pack the same punch as stir fried spinach. For one thing, there's a volume issue. Many greens cook down to a much smaller amount than they started out. It takes several cups of raw spinach, for instance, to give you a half- to a whole-cup serving of cooked. The same is true with Swiss chard or beet greens. The other key is degree of darkness. The darker the green color, the more chlorophyll, and the more beneficial nutrients. Broccoli, collards, and kale are thus richer in nutrients that iceberg lettuce or Napa cabbage.

CHLOROPHYLL, ENERGY, AND CALMNESS

Green plants contain chlorophyll, the molecule that gives them their rich color. As we have just learned, the darker the green of a leafy plant, the more chlorophyll, magnesium, protein, and B vitamins it has. Broccoli, collards, and kale are thus richer in chlorophyll and nutrients than iceberg lettuce or Napa cabbage. Even more nutrient-dense are the concentrated green food supplements such as wild blue-green algae, chlorella, barley grass, and wheat grass, among others, which you can purchase at a health food store.

According to Paul Pitchford in his book, *Healing with Whole Foods*, green is the "master color," meaning it can benefit all patterns of imbalance or conditions. Chlorophyll incorporates the essential energizing, yet at the same time calming, mineral magnesium into its center.

The calm, centered serenity of true balance, a state in which we are happy, mentally clear, healthy, and energized, requires a balance of minerals. Perhaps the most common mineral shortage that erodes our sense of balance, as well as our health, is magnesium, the mineral that forms the center of the chlorophyll molecule in dark green leafy vegetables. Magnesium is a yin nutrient; it helps quench heat-producing oxidation reactions and inflammation (including headaches and PMS), calm our energy, regulate our heart beat and blood pressure, stabilize our blood-sugar levels and moods, and build strong bones. The mineral magnesium is involved in more than 300 enzymatic reactions in the body. Magnesium-rich diets are thought to protect against PMS, diabetes, asthma, chronic fatigue, bone loss, high blood pressure, and heart attacks. A 1978 study showed an inverse relationship between magnesium in drinking water and heart attacks. The more magnesium people get in their water and food, the less their risk of heart disease.[102]

I can tell almost immediately when someone will benefit by adding magnesium to his or her diet. Karina, a forty-five-year-old client of mine, sits rigid in the chair across from me, her brow furrowed. Her concerns about our session, her weight, her work projects, and her problems with her teenage daughter all vie for her attention. She tells me she is tense and agitated most of the time, often tired, has trouble sleeping through the night, and is frequently irritable. She suffers from constipation from time to time and from headaches regularly. She also craves chocolate. These are all signs of magnesium deficiency. As soon as Karina begins eating cooked spinach, broccoli, or other leafy greens each day, plus taking a magnesium supplement, she relaxes, her cravings diminish, sleep becomes easier, and her bowel habits normalize. She tells me, "Even though the stresses of my life are basically the same, I feel calmer, better able to cope."

A 1994 US Department of Agriculture study of 37,785 individuals found only 25 percent had magnesium intakes at or greater than the recommended daily allowance. A review of the scientific studies shows our intake of magnesium is only a fraction of the RDA.[103] With processing, and the majority of our food is highly processed, 75 percent of magnesium in food is lost. But let's say you're getting plenty of greens and other foods rich in magnesium. Did you know eating excess fat, sugar, or phosphate-containing foods such as soft drinks and meats, as well as drinking alcohol and coping with stress, increases our need for magnesium?

THE REAL THING VERSUS VITAMIN PILLS

Even though researchers have identified hundreds of powerful disease-fighting nutrients, other substances in foods—a host of other life-imbuing factors—still remain a mystery to us. Researchers at the USDA Jean Mayer Human Nutrition Research Center at Tufts University in Boston show fruits and vegetables supply antioxidant nutrients other than the vitamins and minerals we've been able to isolate and put into pills, nutrients perhaps more important in providing cancer protection than the current key players that we have already identified, vitamin C, E, and carotenoids. Perhaps only through observation of the effects of different foods will we fully understand their potential for health and healing. In the meantime, don't rely on vitamin pills—eat your vegetables and fruits every day. Choose seasonal fruits and vegetables as much as possible, focusing on those best for your particular body pattern, and enjoy.

CHOOSING VEGETABLES AND FRUITS FOR YOUR PATTERN

Vegetables and Fruits for a Heat Pattern (or for Summer)

Vegetables and fruits are the most powerful foods to use in cooling a pattern of excess heat, including high blood pressure, high cholesterol, and a tendency toward anger and restlessness. TCM and Western research reinforce one another in this area. Fruits and vegetables provide therapeutic levels of potassium, magnesium, antioxidants, and other phytochemicals—critical nutrients in reducing risk of stroke, heart attack, and cancer. They can also keep us cool on a hot summer day.

In general, green, blue, and purple vegetables and fruits tend to be more cooling than red, orange, or yellow foods. The most cooling vegetables include cucumbers and most leafy greens, especially spinach, broccoli, watercress, Swiss chard, lettuce, and Napa cabbage. Other cooling vegetables include raw celery and snow peas, as well as cooked eggplant and zucchini. Among the most cooling fruits are honeydew melon, blueberries, and kiwi fruits. All vegetables and fruits are more cooling raw than when cooked.

The bitter flavor, in TCM, is considered the most cooling flavor and thus benefits a pattern of heat. It also helps eliminate dampness. Many leafy greens are bitter, including romaine lettuce, dandelion greens, arugula, asparagus, lettuce, and alfalfa sprouts.

Salty foods can be cooling or heating. Small amounts of salt tend to be more cooling. Sea vegetables, plants rich in sodium, magnesium, and calcium, are particularly cooling and moistening. They have therapeutic value for those at risk of heart disease and those with other signs of heat. Adding certain salty flavorings to vegetable dishes also helps balance heat (as well as cold). Cooling salty seasonings include soy sauce, sea salt, and miso soup. Those with high blood pressure as part of their heat pattern should use caution with salty condiments.

A few pungent vegetables and spices are cooling or neutral and benefit a pattern of heat, especially when accompanied by dampness. These include peppermint, marjoram, radish, daikon radish, and kohlrabi. The spicy, pungent flavor of chilies, garlic, onions, chives, leeks, and other members of the onion family are very warming. Too many of these foods can aggravate a pattern of heat.

When lightly cooked, especially in broth or other liquids, vegetables provide a refreshingly yin, soothing, cooling quality to the body. If stir fried, deep fried, or roasted at high heat, especially with warming spices, the same vegetables become yang, stimulating, and relatively warming. Large amounts of garlic, dried ginger, cinnamon, black pepper, or hot chilies are too warming for most people with signs of heat and are best minimized or avoided.

VEGETABLE IDEAS FOR A HEAT PATTERN (OR FOR SUMMER)

Avoid raw vegetables if you have symptoms of indigestion, gas, or bloating.

Broth-steamed Napa cabbage with sweet potatoes, soy sauce, and toasted black sesame seeds

Steamed broccoli with lemon juice, lemon zest, sea salt, and cracked white pepper

Swiss chard sautéed in canola oil with raisins

Snow peas and water chestnuts sautéed in canola oil with rice wine, and mushroom flavored soy sauce

Eggplant and summer squash brushed with olive oil, sprinkled with sea salt and grilled

Salad greens with cucumber, tomato, and feta cheese (made from sheep's milk), drizzled with olive oil and balsamic vinegar

Spinach sautéed in olive oil, seasoned with lemon juice, and a pinch of nutmeg

"Creamy" watercress soup (purée cooked watercress, wakame leaves, and sea salt with well cooked white beans in chicken or vegetable broth and season with sea salt and white pepper)

Romaine lettuce, tomatoes, and alfalfa sprouts, and red beans with "creamy" avocado dressing (avocado, goat yogurt, lemon juice, sea salt and white pepper, combined and puréed)

Vegetable soup (potato, corn, carrots, celery, thyme, and white pepper)

Vegetables and Fruits for a Cold Pattern (or for Winter)

Even though vegetables and fruits are generally cooler than meats and oily foods, they are essential to achieving balance and peak health even for those with a cold pattern, or on a cold winter day. Any vegetable or fruit can be warmed through cooking and warming seasonings. Sautéing, stir frying, grilling, roasting, and baking plus seasoning with garlic, cinnamon, ginger, or black pepper are excellent ways of adding warmth to your favorite vegetables or fruits.

The pungent flavor of some vegetables is particularly helpful in warming the body and circulating energy, blood, and vital energy, or Qi. Many pungent vegetables, herbs, and spices are warming and therefore beneficial to damp and cold conditions. They help stimulate a sluggish or slow digestion. Warming, pungent vegetables and spices include mustard greens, kale, broccoli rabe, cabbage, parsley, chilies, rosemary, scallions, onions, garlic, leeks, cinnamon, cloves, ginger, black pepper, cayenne, turmeric, fennel, horseradish, and nutmeg.

The sweet flavor, which encompasses a particularly wide range of foods, including meats, legumes, many grains, and some vegetables, also tends to be relatively warming, as well as moistening. Some fruits are even warming. The best vegetable choices for a pattern of cold include sweet-tasting winter squashes such as butternut, acorn, kobocha, delicata, and banana squash. You can bring out their potential for deeply warming the tissues of the body by baking them with butter and cinnamon, olive oil and garlic, or toasted sesame oil and toasted sesame seeds.

In general, red, orange, or yellow (yang colors) vegetables and fruits are more warming than blue, green, or purple (yin colors) foods. Deep orange squashes, parsnips, and red peppers are more warming than eggplant, spinach, or cucumbers.

Although most fruits are refreshing and cooling, a number of fruits are actually warming and, in small amounts, can benefit those with a pattern of cold. If dampness in the form of fluid retention, abdominal bloating, or excess body fat are present, however, fruits should be used with caution. Warming fruits include cherries, apricots, peaches, nectarines, dates, coconut, and pineapple. In cases of abdominal bloating, diarrhea, or gas, however, all raw fruits should be avoided or minimized.

VEGETABLE IDEAS FOR A COLD PATTERN (OR FOR WINTER)

Broccoli rabe sautéed with garlic in olive oil with sea salt and cracked black pepper

Collard greens boiled in chicken broth, then sautéed in canola oil and sprinkled with toasted mustard seeds

Root vegetables oven-roasted with garlic-infused olive oil and sea salt (carrots, rutabagas, turnips and parsnips)

Onions and mushrooms grilled in canola oil with cumin seeds

Shredded kale with scallions and garlic sautéed in olive oil

Stir-fried asparagus and parsnips with ginger and oyster sauce

Mustard greens sautéed in olive oil with balsamic vinegar

Baked winter squash topped with toasted sesame oil and toasted sesame seeds

Purée of greens soup (boiled mustard and turnip greens, kale, and onion with peeled celery root cubes in beef broth, seasoned with sea salt and black pepper, and puréed until creamy.)

Red cabbage braised in red wine spiced with cinnamon, whole cloves, ginger, and olive oil

Vegetables and Fruits for a Damp Pattern

Vegetables are a vital food for drying dampness and therefore for eliminating excess body fat, masses such as cysts and tumors, and fluid retention. Vegetables are the best foods to reach for when you have sinus mucous or a congested, toxic intestine (marked by sluggish digestion with poor elimination or constipation, both signs of dampness). The fiber and nutrient content as well as the fast-growing nature of many vegetables correlates with their ability to move Qi, our vital energy, and thus the accumulated fat, fluids, or swellings associated with energy that stops circulating. In Western terms, the Qi-moving, damp-dispelling properties of vegetables are a result of their being low in calories and high in fiber. Low-calorie, high-fiber, Qi-moving, damp-dispelling qualities are those best for fat-burning, weight loss, and protection against cancer and heart attacks—all conditions associated with dampness.

Bitter or pungent vegetables are the most beneficial in drying a pattern of dampness. These include broccoli rabe, watercress, dandelion greens, turnip, daikon radish, radishes, celery, cabbage, kohlrabi, asparagus, pumpkin, and scallion. When dampness is accompanied by cold, the spicy pungent foods—chilies, ginger, cayenne, black pepper, garlic, onions, leeks, chives—can be increased. When accompanied by heat, the cooling pungent and bitter foods, including peppermint, marjoram, radish, and celery, can be added for balance.

The energizing, diuretic action of almost all dark leafy greens make them particularly helpful in drying patterns of dampness. Two exceptions, however, are spinach and Swiss chard, which tend to be moistening.

To help reduce dampness, vegetables are best baked, stir fried, sautéed with very little oil, or cooked into clear soups. Heavy use of oils, butter, or salt can leave vegetables more damp-producing.

Sweet vegetables, including potatoes, winter squash, sweet potatoes, and yams can produce dampness, especially when overeaten or combined with meats, beans, or other protein foods. They can be beneficial, however, seasoned with pungent herbs, including anise, fennel seed, mustard seed, or cumin, and when used as a replacement for grains, especially pasta or bread. Fruits, with their sweet nature, tend to produce dampness. Tropical fruits such as pineapple, papaya, dates, bananas, and mangoes are particularly damp-producing and should be avoided by those with signs of dampness.

Food combinations can also affect the tendency of meals to be damp or drying. Fruits eaten at the same time as vegetables, sugars, or meats tend to produce dampness more readily than fruits eaten alone as a snack. Fruit-sugar combinations such as jam and jellies, pies, and other fruit desserts are particularly damp-producing.

Starchy vegetables, including carrots, beets, potatoes, parsnips, and winter squash, can be damp-producing when consumed at the same meal as meat, fish, poultry, beans, or other protein foods. Starchy vegetables are best for a damp condition when served with succulent vegetables such as cauliflower, brussels sprouts, broccoli, or turnips.

The ideal eating plan for drying dampness is one that focuses on cooked, non-starchy vegetables, lean poultry, fish, and small amounts of drying grains such as rice and rye. Fruits, if eaten at all, should be eaten alone, between meals as snacks.

VEGETABLE SUGGESTIONS FOR A DAMP PATTERN

Grilled asparagus with lemon juice and turmeric

Boiled pumpkin with snow peas, sprinkled with roasted pumpkin seeds

Shiitake mushrooms and Napa cabbage sautéed in small amount of olive oil seasoned with cracked pepper

Radicchio, portobello mushrooms, and summer squash, brushed with olive oil and grilled

Bok choy, turnips, and carrots stir fried in canola oil with minced fresh ginger

Julienned daikon and watercress seasoned with toasted sesame oil, rice vinegar and tamari sauce

Fennel and fresh corn on the cob grilled on open barbecue

Broccoli rabe, boiled, drizzled with olive oil, and sprinkled with toasted mustard seeds

Broth-steamed broccoli and turnips with cumin

Vegetable soup (celery, corn, turnips, snow peas, zucchini, oregano, marjoram, thyme, and cracked pepper)

Vegetables and Fruits for a Dry Pattern

Although vegetables can have a diuretic effect by ridding the body of excess fluids, they also provide minerals and other nutrients necessary to moisten and calm the thirsty pattern of dryness. The yin nature of most vegetables, especially when combined with essential-fat rich foods such as fatty fish, seeds, or beneficial oils, provides a moistening quality that helps to soothe the irritability, restless sleep, dry flaky skin, and dry throat and mouth common in a pattern of dryness. Dark green leafy vegetables—rich in magnesium, essential oils, and fiber—also help even out blood sugar and thus reduce sugar cravings typical in those with a pattern of dryness.

The sweet and salty flavored vegetables tend to be the best choices for moistening dryness. Sea vegetables, including wakame, kelp, and dulse, are among the foods richest in moistening salts, iodine, magnesium, and calcium—yin, fluid-building minerals. They are ideal cooked into soups, bean dishes, rice, or stir fried vegetable dishes. Sweet vegetables, including winter squash, carrots, parsnips, and beets, are also helpful in restoring yin fluids.

Moistening vegetables also include spinach, Swiss chard, mushrooms, green beans, Napa cabbage, and asparagus. All vegetables can be helpful to balancing a pattern of dryness, because they contain moisture. When cooked with small amounts of salt and oils, vegetables are better able to convey their moistening quality to body tissues.

Fruits best able to provide a balanced moistening effect include bananas, pears, figs, and avocados. Because blood-sugar control is so important in a pattern of dryness, fruit juices and dried fruits (both concentrated source of sugar) are best avoided. They can cause blood-sugar levels to skyrocket, ultimately rebounding to low blood-sugar levels and thus precipitating cravings for more sugars.

VEGETABLE SUGGESTIONS FOR A DRY PATTERN

Green beans boiled in chicken broth and drizzled with olive oil and sea salt

Red and gold beets, brushed with olive oil, then oven-roasted with sea salt

Carrot soup, seasoned with dill weed and sunflower seeds, topped with dollop of goat yogurt

Eggplant, broccoli, and water chestnuts cooked in sauce of coconut milk and curry

Stir fried Napa cabbage, carrots and mushrooms with oyster sauce

Sweet potatoes, boiled, then sautéed with spinach and garlic

Swiss chard sautéed in olive oil with toasted pine nuts

Spinach, mushroom and goat cheese omelet

Stir fried mixed vegetables, tofu and black bean sauce

Acorn squash brushed with olive oil, sprinkled with sea salt and baked

---

93. Koletzko., B. et al., "Pesticides in Dietary Foods for Infnats and Young Children," *Arch Dis Child* 80 (1999): 91–92.
94. Dich, Jan, and Kirsten Wiklund, "Prostate Cancer in Pesticide Applicators in Swedish Agriculture," *The Prostate* 34 (1998): 100–12.
95. Dorgan, J. F., "Serum Organochlorino Pesticides and PCB's and Breast Cancer Risk: Results from a Prospective Analysis (USA)," *Cancer Causes Control* (1999): 101–11.
96. *Circulation* (September 22, 1998).
97. Weil, Andrew, MD, *8 Weeks to Optional Health*. NY: Alfred Knopf, (1997).
98. Hall, J. and Solehdin, F. "Folic Acid for the Prevention of Congenital Anomalies," *European Journal of Pediatrics* 157 (1998):445–50.
99. Ford E.S. et. al., "Serum Folate and Chronic Disease Risk: Findings from a Cohort of United StatesAdults," *International Journal of Epidemiology* 27(1998): 592–98
100,101,102. Lewis C.J. et. al., "Estimated Folate Intakes: Data Updated to Reflect Food Fortification, Increased Bioavailability, and Dietary Supplement Use," *American Journal of Clinical Nutrition* 70(1999):198–207.
103. Weil, Andrew, MD, *8 Weeks to Optimal Health*. New York: Alfred Knopf, (1997).

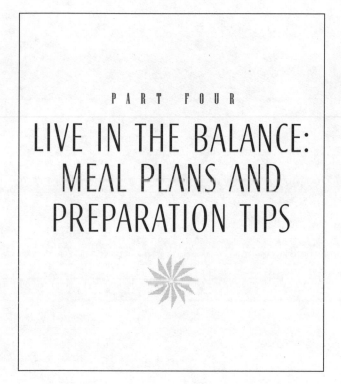

PART FOUR

LIVE IN THE BALANCE: MEAL PLANS AND PREPARATION TIPS

15

EATING GUIDELINES AND
FOOD PORTIONS FOR
OPTIMUM HEALTH

The guidelines given here are appropriate for all patterns and will benefit those who feel healthy as well as those with signs of imbalance. This lifestyle and eating plan helps prevent disease and promote optimum health, peak energy, and ideal weight. Each of its elements is designed to strengthen spleen Qi, or digestion, which is critical to the health of all your organs, to boosting immunity, to maintaining ideal weight, and to having energy. The Qi and essences extracted from digestion provide vitality, warmth, blood, and fluids for the sustenance of all tissues. Strengthening the spleen is the first step toward optimizing health and normalizing body weight. (See chapter three for more about spleen Qi.)

Unlike most diet programs, which give precise measurements for calories and portions, the quantities here are provided as guidelines only. Your long-term health depends on your ability to listen to your body's subtle cues as to what and how much to eat. Naturally thin people don't weigh out a portion of rice. They have an inherent ability to know when their bodies have had enough. Once you achieve balance, your body's wisdom will let you know when you've had the right amount of noodles. You'll be able to push away the plate of bread and to luxuriate in one bite of flourless chocolate cake and say "perfect," without the need to anesthetize yourself by eating the whole thing. On the other hand, you may feel like having six ounces of salmon at dinner one night and the next night want little more than a bite of fish or chicken.

This program avoids calorie counting as a way to determine portions. In the Asian system of evaluating foods, the "build up" and "break down" qualities of foods can be more useful concepts than calories. Meat, dairy products, refined sugars, and wheat are "build up" foods. They can put weight on us more readily than vegetables, seafood, or rice can, regardless of their caloric value. In addition, certain fats help stimulate metabolism and are therefore fat-burning. Omega-3 fats, found in fish and certain seeds and their oils, actually help burn fat. Saturated and hydrogenated fats, from margarine, vegetable shortening, bacon, steak, and butter, are, on the other hand, linked with obesity; they also increase your need for the fat-burning properties of essential fats. The bottom line is you can eat more food (and calories) and still lose weight if you're choosing more "break down" or fat-burning foods than "build-up" foods.

Perhaps just as important as what foods you eat is when you eat them. One of the healthiest practices and easiest ways to lose or maintain weight is to eat lightly at the end of the day. The people of most other countries have figured this out already and take their heaviest meal at midday and their lightest meal at night.

In the general guidelines below, a range of portion sizes is given for each category of food. You will need to determine the amount that's right for you by taking into consideration a variety of factors, including your hunger level, body pattern, activity level, age, sex, height, frame, metabolism, lean body mass, and other food choices. The longer you eat truly balanced meals, the more precise your body wisdom in determining portions will become. To begin to learn your ideal portions and be happy with them, try practicing the following five steps at meal times:

1. Before you sit down to eat, take a moment to relax. Sit quietly and close your eyes. Shift your attention from your thoughts to your body and feelings. Allow yourself to form a picture of how much food is appropriate for you.

2. Begin to experience a feeling of gratitude for your food. Savor it with your eyes and inhale the aromas deeply. This begins the process of digestion and facilitates the ultimate feeling of satisfaction.
3. If you tend to overeat at meals, have a cup of clear soup before eating to begin the process of feeling satisfied sooner.
4. Eat slowly. Remember it takes twenty minutes for your brain to get the message that your stomach is full.
5. Leave the table and any remaining food before you feel completely full. If you feel hungry within a few hours after eating, you may need more essential fat at meals or you may need to eat more. You should be able to make it four to six hours before your next meal.

General Guidelines for Optimum Health and Balance

1. Engage in aerobic activity thirty minutes to one hour daily. Choose from walking, jogging, hiking, bicycling, dancing, swimming, aerobic machines, or any other similar activity that you enjoy.
2. Adopt a daily practice of relaxation (meditation, yoga, T'ai chi, quiet reflection). Spend more time in awareness activities or inner reflection during winter.
3. At meals, in particular, allow time for relaxation, and always eat in a calm environment. Don't work, read, or engage in frustrating or anxiety-provoking conversation while eating.
4. Chew every bite from twenty to fifty times.
5. Eat lightly. Don't overeat.
6. Eat three light meals per day, with 25 percent of food in the morning, 50 percent at midday, and 25 percent in the evening. Don't overeat at night.
7. Include two and a half to four cups of seasonal vegetables per day, the majority (75 to 95 percent) lightly cooked. Choose more root vegetables and winter squashes in fall and winter, more leafy greens, snap peas, and spinach in spring, and more summer squashes, tomatoes, eggplant, and corn in summer. During the summer, eat more raw vegetables; during the winter, eat more cooked vegetables. Include one half to one cup cooked seasonal leafy green vegetables daily. Have more salads in spring and summer and more cooked, warming greens in winter.

8. Choose one to three fresh, seasonal fruits per day (more in spring and summer, fewer in winter). Have more cooked fruits in winter.

9. Include well-cooked whole grains, breads, pasta, crackers, or other whole grain foods at each meal. Eat more cooling grains, such as millet, in summer and more warming grains, such as buckwheat, in winter. A serving size is one half to one-and-a-half cups of cooked whole grains or pasta; one to two slices of bread; one to two corn tortillas; or three to five crackers.

10. Include protein two to three times per day (more in winter than in summer). Vary your choices; include more seafood, legumes, tofu, nuts, and seeds in spring and summer and more poultry, red meat, and eggs in fall and winter. A serving size is two to five ounces of seafood, meats, or poultry; one to two eggs; two to three tablespoons of nuts or seeds; one half to one cup beans, peas, or lentils; or five to eight ounces of tofu.

11. Include an essential fat–rich food each day. Choose from cold-water fatty fish, pumpkin seeds, flaxseeds, flaxseed oil, hemp seeds, hemp seed oil, canola oil, or soy products.

12. Include foods from each of the five flavors (sour, salty, sweet, pungent, and bitter) and the five colors (green, red/orange, dark [black/brown], white, and yellow) whenever possible.

13. Take a multivitamin and mineral supplement with one or more meals each day.

14. Drink only small amounts of liquids with meals.

15. Limit refined sugars (sucrose, fructose, corn syrup, high-fructose corn syrup, maltose, rice syrup, fruit-juice sweeteners, molasses, honey) to less than a tablespoon per day.

16. Avoid or limit alcohol to one to two drinks per day.

17. Avoid cold foods and drinks (iced water, cold drinks, ice cream, and frozen desserts).

16

MEAL SUGGESTIONS AND COOKING TIPS FOR REDUCING SIGNS OF HEAT AND FOR SUMMER COMFORT

The following cooking suggestions and meal ideas can be helpful in cooling signs of excess heat. They can also be helpful on hot days or anytime you're looking for a way to cool down—physically or emotionally. Cooling meals and cooking methods can be helpful during highly stressful or frustrating periods in your life. If I wind up working long hours or am working hard to meet a deadline, I may feel more irritable than usual, and know I need to reach for more vegetables and grains, along with tofu, beans, or poached fish to soothe my body and calm my nerves.

As you will recall from chapter six, a pattern of excess heat may include signs such as a red face, a tendency to feel too warm and an aversion to hot weather, a voracious appetite and huge thirst, restlessness and irritability, high blood pressure and high cholesterol levels, headaches, and sometimes dream-disturbed sleep.

The ideal eating plan for such a pattern includes drinking generous amounts of cool water plus following a diet rich in lightly cooked and raw vegetables as well as cooling fruits. These foods are supplemented with cooling grains, some fish, beans, and soy products. A vegetarian diet with lots of raw and some cooked vegetables will most quickly remedy a pattern of excess heat. Overuse of alcohol, tobacco, meat, saturated fats, fried foods, hydrogenated vegetable oil, or spicy foods, including garlic, ginger, cinnamon, cayenne, and chilies, can worsen a heat pattern.

Guidelines to Reduce Heat or Cool off in Summertime

1. Drink cool bottled or purified water throughout the day (eight to twelve glasses).
2. Incorporate light, pleasing exercise (golf; walking, especially in nature; swimming; or yoga) into your life daily.
3. Include a regular practice of relaxation or awareness exercise (mediation, yoga, T'ai chi).
4. Include two and a half to five cups of lightly cooked and raw vegetables per day (50 to 60 percent raw), including lettuce, spinach, watercress, and other bitter leafy greens.
5. Include two servings of protein per day, preferably from the following: seafood, tofu, soy products, or beans. Limit beef. Avoid lamb.
6. Choose two to three servings of cooling or moistening whole grains per day, such as corn, rye, millet, or wild rice.
7. Include two to three pieces of cooling fruits per day, including kiwi, berries, melon, grapefruit, apples, blueberries, bananas, or pears.
8. Increase bitter and sour foods and decrease sweet and pungent foods. Balance each of the flavors.

 NOTE *The "sweet" flavor refers not only to empty sweets such as ice cream, cookies, and candy, but also to full sweets, including poultry, meats, seafood, fruit, root vegetables, and whole grains.*

9. Balance cooling foods with very small amounts of warming seasonings (garlic, ginger, and so on).

Breakfast Suggestions to Reduce Heat
1. Cooked millet with plain yogurt or soy milk and ground flax seeds
   Fresh blueberries

Cooling herb tea blend or water (see p. 245)

NOTE *Flaxseeds are an excellent source of essential oils, fiber, and protein. When added to hot cereals, they provide a nutty, rich, grainlike texture and bulk. They are filling, provide moisture, stimulate elimination (alleviate constipation), and help stabilize blood-sugar levels.*

2. Grits with plain yogurt or melted soy cheese
   Fresh grapefruit
   Cooling herb tea blend or water (see p. 245)

TIP: *To flavor hot cereals, use cooling fruits or soy milk. For a delicious, creamy, savory hot cereal, try a mild melted soy cheese or rice cheese. For a traditional sweet flavor in hot cereal or yogurt without using refined sugar, use the naturally sweet herb stevia. Unlike refined sugars, which can disrupt blood sugar levels, stevia helps to stabilize blood sugar. It is 100 to 400 times sweeter than granulated table sugar, depending on how it is extracted. Because stevia is carbohydrate- and calorie-free, it does not trigger fatigue or mood swings, nor does it contribute to diabetes, excess weight gain, elevated blood fat levels, or dental caries like refined sugar can. While refined sugars are inflammatory and heating from a TCM standpoint, stevia is neutral. It is available as a whole leaf extract in either a brown syrup or pale green powder. Although this is the least processed and probably best form of this herb from a health standpoint, some people find it has an unpleasant aftertaste. The refined extract, on the other hand, available in a fine white powder or clear liquid, can easily substitute in flavor for refined sugar in cereals, yogurt or teas. Optimum Nutrition and NuNaturals are among the companies that offer stevia extract through health food stores, including GNC Stores, across the country.*

3. Whole-grain toast with lox or other smoked fish, sliced tomato
   Fresh pear
   Cooling herb tea blend or water (see p. 245)
4. Whole-grain toast with soy cream cheese, sliced cucumber, sliced tomato
   Fresh blackberries
   Cooling herb tea blend or water (see p. 245)
5. Breakfast burrito: pinto beans, diced tomatoes, lettuce, and avocado slices wrapped in a whole-wheat flour tortilla or corn tortilla
   Honeydew melon
   Cooling herb tea blend or water (see p. 245)
6. Spinach and mushroom omelet (use two whites per whole egg)

Rye or rice toast with omega-rich spread
Fresh watermelon or strawberries
Cooling herb tea blend or water (see p. 245)

Lunch Suggestions to Reduce Heat

1. Mung bean and vegetable soup
   Boiled new potatoes with olive oil, chopped parsley, lemon juice, sea salt, and white pepper
   Green salad with radishes, bean sprouts, and cherry tomatoes (dress with olive oil, lemon juice, and fresh or dried marjoram)
   Sourdough bread with olive oil, cucumber, and tomato slices
2. Green salad of mixed lettuces, lima beans, cucumbers, sliced tomatoes (dress with olive oil, herbs, and lemon juice), topped with crumbled aged goat cheese
   Brown or black rice with chopped olives and fresh basil
3. Fresh crab (with cocktail sauce or lemon juice) on bed of lettuce
   Swiss chard or spinach sautéed in olive oil, flavored with sea salt, lemon juice, and white pepper
   Carrot sticks
   Dill pickle
   Whole-grain bread with pat of omega-rich spread
4. Three-bean salad and marinated artichokes over mixed lettuce greens
   Grilled vegetables (eggplant, carrots, and squash with olive oil and kelp or dulse sprinkles)
   Sauerkraut

 TIP *If cooking beans from scratch, add kombu, wakame, or other sea vegetables to cooking water to cool the body and moisten signs of dryness (build yin fluids) as well as reduce problems with gas.*

   Whole-wheat pita bread with hummus and cucumber slices
5. Vegetable-tofu (or tempeh) stir fry (carrots, snow peas, water chestnuts, bean sprouts, tofu or tempeh pieces, and soaked hijiki

seaweed, lightly stir fried in canola oil and flavored with sesame oil and tamari sauce)

Seaweed salad

Steamed rice with toasted sesame seeds

Dinner Suggestions to Reduce Heat

1. Fresh cracked crab on bed of baby lettuces with cucumber slices and vinaigrette dressing

    Sautéed broccoli with lemon and anchovy

    Whole-grain sourdough bread with hummus spread

    (Vegetarian suggestion: Substitute garbanzo beans and kidney beans for crab)

2. Grilled halibut filet (marinate twenty minutes in soy sauce, miso paste, rice vinegar, a few drops stevia liquid, and small amount grated ginger) on bed of raw watercress and raw sliced daikon radishes

    Stir fried bok choy and water chestnuts with soy sauce

    Steamed black rice

    (Vegetarian suggestion: Substitute grilled tofu for halibut)

3. Split pea soup with cauliflower and carrots, sprinkled with pumpkin seeds

    Mixed green salad with sliced pears, crumbled goat cheese, drizzle of olive oil and lemon juice, seasoned with sea salt and cracked white pepper

    Whole-grain bread with tofu cream cheese and cucumber and tomato slices

    (Vegetarian suggestion: Substitute grilled marinated tempeh for salmon)

4. Turkey salad (lettuce, white, skinless turkey pieces, julienned carrots, and radishes, dressed with a small amount olive oil, lemon juice, fresh dill, and kelp or dulse sprinkles)

    Baked potato topped with vegetable broth and plain yogurt

    Spinach and shiitake mushrooms lightly sautéed in olive oil

    (Vegetarian suggestion: Substitute garbanzo beans or soy

"turkey" for roasted turkey)

5. Grilled tofu or tempeh (marinate in miso paste, tamari sauce, a few drops stevia, and a small amount of garlic)

> Mixed raw salad greens with kidney beans, blanched cauliflower, and roasted red peppers, canola oil, lemon juice, dried tarragon, sea salt and white pepper
>
> Whole-wheat or rice noodles cooked with snow peas and fresh basil leaves in broth, mirin, and soy sauce and topped with toasted sesame seeds

BALANCING SNACKS

apple and sunflower seeds

cucumber and tomato slices, with hummus on whole-grain crackers

soy cheese and pear

baked blue-corn chips with mild bean dip

plain yogurt with lemon juice and stevia

heated tortilla with melted soy Jack cheese and tomato slice

watermelon

COOLING COOKING METHODS

poaching in lemon, water, or broth

steam sautéing

steaming

eating raw vegetables and fruits

braising

choose primarily cold, cooling, and neutral seasonings and flavorings, with a small amount of warming seasonings for balance

NEUTRAL HERBS AND SEASONINGS

chamomile

oat straw

chicory, roasted

rose hips

licorice root (can raise blood pressure)

saffron

miso paste

COOLING HERBS AND SEASONINGS

kudzu (thickener)

lemon/lime juice

   (citrus may aggravate excess

   heat in the stomach)

lemongrass

marjoram

peppermint*

sea salt

sea vegetables (dulse, wakame, hijiki)

tamarind

vegetable broth (when made with cooling vegetables)

* cold herbs

COOLING TEAS AND BEVERAGES

catnip

chicory

chrysanthemum fkower

dandelion leaves and root

green tea

hibiscus

lemon balm

nettles

passionflower

peppermint

red clover blossoms

red raspberry leaf

soy milk

Several herbs can be combined to make a tasty balancing blend. For a cooling tea blend, combine several cooling herbs with a small addition of a neutral or warming herb. For each cup of tea, pour boiling water over about a tablespoon of herb mix and let steep 3–5 minutes. Try a combination of red clover, peppermint, lemon balm, and chamomile with a pinch of orange peel.

17

MEAL SUGGESTIONS AND COOKING TIPS FOR REDUCING SIGNS OF COLD AND FOR WINTER WARMTH

The following cooking suggestions and meal ideas can be helpful in balancing signs of cold or when the climate turns cold. They are also helpful if you want a more focused and assertive quality of energy. As you will recall from chapter five, a cold pattern may include signs such as a pale complexion, a tendency to feel chilled or cold and an aversion to cold weather, anemia, depression, fatigue, and loose stools. Warming foods can also be helpful on winter days, or anytime you're looking for a way to warm up or to feel stronger or more fortified emotionally. Since a cold pattern is a yin condition, the remedy is to increase yang foods. Yang foods can also energize you for a day of physical activity or for an important presentation or negotiation.

The ideal eating plan focuses on cooked high-protein foods, including chicken, beef, red-fleshed fish, and lamb, along with onions, garlic, and other warming foods and spices. Vegetables are best cooked using plenty of warming seasonings. Raw fruits, salads, and cold foods should be avoided or reduced. It is difficult to warm a pattern of cold with a vegetarian diet. If you're a vegetarian and you have signs of cold, prepare your meals with generous amounts of warming seasonings, including cinnamon, ginger, mustard seeds, cumin, turmeric, curry, and garlic.

Guidelines for Reducing Cold Signs and Stimulating Performance Energy

1. Include twenty minutes or more of daily aerobic exercise. Choose from walking, jogging, bicycling, dancing, aerobics classes, exercise machines, or other invigorating, enjoyable activity.
2. Incorporate strength training into your daily exercise program: weights, nautilus, sit-ups, pull-ups.
3. Include two and a half to four cups of cooked, neutral or warming vegetables per day, seasoned with warming spices such as garlic, onions, turmeric, cayenne, and/or black pepper.
4. Include three servings of protein per day, preferably from the following: red meat—especially lamb—chicken, turkey, pheasant, red-fleshed fish, eel, shrimp, lake or stream fish. If you are a vegetarian or want meatless meals, focus on black beans or fava beans cooked with cumin, fennel seed, garlic, ginger, or other warming spices, and include regular use of walnuts, almonds, or pine nuts. Avoid tofu.
5. Choose three servings of warming whole grains per day such as quinoa, buckwheat, basmati rice, or oats. Avoid wheat.
6. Increase full sweet and pungent foods and decrease bitter and sour foods. Balance each of the flavors.

 TIP *The "sweet" flavor refers not only to empty sweets such as ice cream, cookies, and candy, but also to full sweets, including poultry, meats, seafood, fruit, root vegetables, and whole grains.*

7. Balance a diet of primarily warming foods with small amounts of cooling seasonings.

Breakfast Suggestions to Increase Warmth
1. Hot oatmeal with cinnamon, nutmeg, and walnuts
   Lean chicken sausage (choose walnuts or almond cheese if vegetarian)

Warming tea or grain beverage (see p. 252)
2. Cooked quinoa with melted almond cheese
   Turkey sausage (choose soy sausage or almonds if vegetarian)
   Warming tea or grain beverage (see p. 252)

TIP *To flavor hot cereals, use walnuts, almonds, and/or cooked warming fruits, plus cinnamon or nutmeg. For a delicious, creamy, savory hot cereal, try a mild melted almond or goat's milk cheese. For a more traditional sweet flavor in hot cereal, use brown-rice syrup, molasses, barley-malt syrup, or maple syrup. The naturally sweet herb stevia adds sweetness without adding calories, plus it helps to stabilize blood sugar. It is 100 to 400 times sweeter than sugar, depending on how it is extracted. I prefer the whole-leaf extract, which comes as a brown syrup. It is neutral and can be used by all patterns. Just six to eight drops will sweeten a bowl of hot cereal or a ten-ounce glass glass of lemonade. It can also be used to sweeten a cooking sauce.*

3. Sprouted mixed grain and seeded toast
   Lox or other smoked fish, onion, and capers
   Warming tea or grain beverage (see p. 252)
   (Vegetarian suggestion: Substitute almond cheese for fish)
4. Scrambled eggs with parsley, chives, and smoked salmon
   Sprouted grain bread with butter or omega-rich spread
   Warming tea or grain beverage (see p. 252)
   (Vegetarian suggestion: Substitute leeks for smoked salmon)
5. Over easy egg(s)
   Steamed basmati rice with scallions and toasted sesame oil
   Toasted black sesame seeds
   Warming tea or grain beverage (see p. 252)

Lunch Suggestions to Increase Warmth
1. Curried prawns (cook cauliflower, onions, broccoli pieces, parsnips, and jumbo prawns, in coconut milk, curry paste or powder, sea salt, and chicken broth)
   Steamed basmati rice or rice noodles
   Hot miso soup

(Vegetarian suggestion: Substitute lentils and fresh whole peas for prawns)

2. Chicken-ginger rice soup (choose a basic recipe using whole chicken. Add coarsely minced ginger, diced onions, parsley, basmati rice, and peas)

Sautéed red cabbage and parsnips (season with celery seeds or curry powder)

Pickled vegetable

(Vegetarian suggestion: Black bean and rice soup, seasoned with onion, cumin, cayenne, and black pepper)

3. Ginger-beef vegetable stir-fry (stir fry thinly sliced flank steak or London broil in minced fresh ginger, with mustard greens, carrots, red peppers, and scallions. Add shrimp-flavored soy sauce, and sake. Simmer until done. Drizzle with a few drops of toasted sesame oil.)

Brown rice noodles with toasted sesame oil and toasted sesame seeds

Dill pickle

(Vegetarian suggestion: Substitute tempeh pieces for beef)

4. Lamb chops with oven-roasted onions, parsnips, and carrots

Sautéed broccoli with garlic and diced olives

Hot quinoa with butter and parsley

Sauerkraut

(Vegetarian suggestion: Add pine nuts to broccoli. For stew: Substitute fava beans stewed with onions, garlic, parsnips, savory, and black pepper)

5. Roasted chicken (season with garlic and fresh rosemary)

Broccoli rabe sautéed in garlic and olive oil, sprinkled with pine nuts

Toasted buckwheat cooked in chicken broth and flavored with olive oil, sea salt, and cracked black pepper, topped with grilled red onions

(Vegetarian suggestion: Omit chicken and replace with tempeh, bite-sized rutabagas, turnips, carrots, and portobello mushrooms roasted in oven with olive oil, garlic, and balsamic vinegar. Top with pine nuts.)

Dinner Suggestions to Increase Warmth

1. Stewed lamb (choose shoulder cut and simmer in red wine, scallions, ginger, cloves, cinnamon, and anise seeds)

   Broth-simmered mustard greens with butter, nutmeg, and black pepper

   Steamed red rice with minced ginger

   (Vegetarian suggestion: Substitute curried lentils with broccoli, peas, and parsnips for lamb.)

2. Grilled ahi filet (marinate twenty minutes in sake, mushroom soy sauce, grated ginger, minced garlic)

   Baked winter squash with black sesame seeds and toasted sesame oil

   Kale blanched in chicken-broth, then sautéed in olive oil with garlic

   Sprouted whole grain bread

   (Vegetarian suggestion: Omit ahi. Add walnut pieces to winter squash. Add freshly shelled fava beans to kale before cooking.)

3. Vegetable beef stew (lean beef pieces stewed in broth, red wine and olive oil with rutabagas, turnips, cabbage, onions, garlic, and savory)

   Quinoa cooked with turnip greens, garlic, olive oil, and cracked black pepper

   (Vegetarian suggestion: Use tempeh instead of beef and use extra onions, savory, and garlic)

4. Chicken-vegetable stew (bake chicken pieces, parsnips, carrots, onions in casserole or clay pot with chicken broth, oyster sauce, and rice wine)

   Kale, shredded and sautéed in olive oil with red pepper flakes and pine nuts

   (Vegetarian suggestion: Substitute tempeh pieces for chicken and use vegetable broth.)

5. Vegetable-salmon stir fry (salmon pieces, asparagus, onions, and red peppers stir fried in canola oil with garlic, a few drops of toasted sesame oil, and fish sauce), topped with toasted sesame seeds

   Steamed red or brown rice

   Miso soup

(Vegetarian suggestion. Omit salmon. Add slivered almonds and use extra ginger and garlic.)

WARMING OR NEUTRAL SNACKS

walnuts	miso soup
almonds	almond cheese and rice crackers
pine nuts	tortilla chips and spicy black-bean dip
chicken soup	smoked salmon
lentil soup	beef jerky
French onion soup	

WARMING COOKING METHODS

grilling	broiling
sautéing	convection oven cooking
baking	pressure cooking
roasting	Avoid raw foods.
barbecuing	

NEUTRAL AND WARMING HERBS AND SEASONINGS

alcohol, wine, sake (in small amounts for cooking)	miso paste
anise seeds	oregano
basil	sage
bay	saffron
caraway seeds	savory
cardamom	sherry
celery seeds	spearmint
chives	sugar (brown and white)
cumin	thyme
dill	turmeric
fenugreek	vegetable broth (made with warming vegetables such as leeks and scallions)

fennel seeds, root

ginger, fresh

vinegar

white peper

HOT HERBS AND SEASONINGS

asafoetida

black pepper

cayenne

chilies (starts out warming but ultimately
becomes cooling)

cinnamon

cloves

garlic

ginger, dried

horseradish

mustard and mustard seeds

nutmeg

red pepper and red-pepper flakes

WARMING TEAS AND BEVERAGES

barley, roasted

black tea

cardamom

cinnamon

ginger, fresh

grain beverages

jasmine tea

oolong tea

orange peel, dried

spearmint

valerian

18

MEAL SUGGESTIONS AND COOKING TIPS FOR REDUCING SIGNS OF DAMPNESS

The following cooking suggestions and meal ideas can be helpful in balancing a pattern of dampness. Minimizing damp foods can also be helpful in humid, muggy, or foggy environments. This plan is particularly effective for weight loss or a slow metabolism. If I gain a few extra pounds from too many rich meals out, I follow this type of plan until I feel I've lost the excess fluids and weight.

As discussed in chapter eight, a pattern of dampness may include signs such as overweight, sinus mucous, abdominal bloating, water retention, fatigue, mental fuzziness, and a feeling of heaviness. The ideal eating plan goes light on portions, and focuses on lightly cooked vegetables, grilled fish, beans, and small amounts of grains, with ideal choices being sprouted grains, amaranth, rye, rice, corn, and other drying grains. Salt is kept to minimum. Pungent herbs, and vegetables, including pepper, cayenne, turmeric, radishes, and turnips, are helpful. Dairy products, soy (including tofu), beef, pork, lamb, sweets, and wheat-containing foods contribute to dampness and should be reduced or eliminated.

Guidelines to Reduce Dampness

1. Include daily aerobic exercise (thirty-five minutes to one hour). Choose from walking, jogging, bicycling, dancing, aerobics classes, exercise machines, or other invigorating enjoyable activity. Keep your living environment dry.

2. Don't overeat. Push away your plate before you feel full. Keep meals simple by not combining too many different foods at one meal and limit water and other beverages with meals.

3. Include two to three cups lightly cooked vegetables per day (limit raw vegetables to 20 percent or less of vegetable intake; less when cold signs are present). Focus on warming vegetables for a damp-cold pattern and more cooling vegetables for a damp-heat pattern.

4. Include two to three servings of protein per day, preferably from the following: beans, peas, lentils, fish, or skinless chicken, pumpkin seeds, eggs/egg whites (limit egg yolks to two per week with signs of damp heat). Limit beef. Avoid lamb and pork.

5. Choose one or two servings daily of sprouted grain bread or drying whole grains, such as basmati rice, wild rice or amaranth. Avoid wheat, buckwheat, sweet rice, sticky rice and pearled barley.

6. Limit raw fruits to one or two seasonal pieces per day as a snack, consumed apart from other foods. Avoid fruits (unless cooked with warming spices) with signs of damp cold.

7. Avoid refined sugar, and cow's milk dairy products, especially together or with other damp foods (for example, pizza and ice cream).

8. Increase bitter (beneficial for damp-heat) flavors and pungent (beneficial for damp-cold) foods while reducing sweet foods. Balance each of the flavors.

TIP *The "sweet" flavor refers not only to empty sweets such as ice cream, cookies, and candy, but also to full sweets, including poultry, meats, seafood, fruit, root vegetables, and whole grains.*

Breakfast Suggestions to Reduce Signs of Dampness with Heat

1. 100–percent rye bread toast
   Chevre cheese or other mild, fresh goat cheese
   Fresh grapefruit
   Green tea
2. Breakfast burrito (pinto beans cooked with a small amount of cumin and sea salt, mixed with chopped lettuce, fresh cilantro in blue corn or yellow corn tortillas)
   Green tea
3. Amaranth cooked with diced green apple
   Pumpkin seeds
   Rice milk (optional)
   Green tea

TIP *To add a creamy flavor and texture to hot cereals, try melting in a small amount of rice cheese (found in health food stores). Other options include roasted pumpkin seeds, raw honey, or the naturally sweet herb stevia. Stevia helps to stabilize blood sugar. It is 100 to 400 times sweeter than sugar, depending on how it is extracted. I prefer the whole-leaf extract, which comes as a brown syrup. It is neutral and can be used by all patterns..*

4. Grits or polenta with melted rice cheese
   Sliced radishes
   Green tea
5. Vegetable omelet (use two whites per whole egg) with blanched broccoli and mushrooms
   100-percent rye or rice toast with omega-rich spread
   Green tea

Lunch Suggestions to Reduce Signs of Dampness with Heat

1. Vegetable stir fry (bean sprouts, broccoli, and red pepper stir fried with small amount canola oil, seasoned with tamari sauce, and miso broth)
   White fish (halibut, perch, snapper, sole) poached in broth, soy sauce, and splash of mirin
   Steamed black or white rice

(Vegetarian suggestion: Omit fish. Add white beans to stir-fry.)

2. Navy-bean or split-pea soup cooked with kombu seaweed

    Salad of raw lettuces, radish slices, mild goat cheese, lemon juice, drizzle of olive oil, sea salt, and cracked white pepper

    Fresh ear of sweet corn, boiled with miso paste

3. Canned white albacore tuna fish mixed with low-fat canola oil mayonnaise, lemon juice, dill pickle pieces, and diced celery (or fresh albacore filet with lemon juice) over bed of romaine lettuce with cracked white pepper

    Rye crackers or sourdough rye bread

    (Vegetarian suggestion: Substitute hard cooked eggs using two whites per whole egg.)

4. Chicken Caesar salad (use white, skinless chicken meat, goat's milk Romano cheese, go light on garlic, and omit croutons)

    Rye or rice bread with omega-rich spread

    (Vegetarian Suggestion: Substitute garbanzo beans for chicken.)

5. Three-bean plus salad (use kidney, mung, garbanzo and green beans)

    Vegetable-rice salad (use steamed, cooled rice and add blanched snap peas, raw radish slices, lemon juice, olive oil, fresh basil, mint and parsley leaves, and cracked white pepper)

    Pickled beets

 TIP *If cooking beans from scratch, add kombu, wakame, or other sea vegetables to cooking water to moisten signs of dryness (build yin fluids) and reduce problems with gas.*

Dinner Suggestions to Reduce Signs of Dampness with Heat

1. Vegetable pasta (use one part dry rice or corn pasta spirals to five parts vegetables; simmer pasta with fresh broccoli pieces, pumpkin pieces, and mushrooms in miso or vegetable broth and lemon juice with fresh basil leaves; time pasta and vegetables so both are done together).

     Small tossed salad with radish slices and avocado dress-
        ing (purée ripe avocado with lemon juice, cilantro, sea
        salt, and white pepper)

2. Steamed white fish with lemon juice and dill weed
     Dandelion greens and water chestnuts braised in small
        amount rice wine and tamari sauce
     Fresh ear sweet corn, boiled
     (Vegetarian suggestion: Substitute vegetable-navy bean
        soup for fish.)

3. Chicken stir fry (skinless white chicken pieces, bok choy, bean
sprouts, and carrots in a small amount of canola oil, miso paste)
     Daikon radish and carrot salad (toss thinly sliced vegeta-
        bles with sesame oil, rice vinegar, and tamari sauce)
     (Vegetarian suggestion: Substitute tempeh for chicken.)

4. Five-bean and vegetable soup (mung, white, aduki, kidney, and
navy beans, onions, mushrooms, celery, and marjoram)
     Broth-steamed cauliflower, and brussels sprouts with
        sesame oil and sesame seeds
     rye bread with omega-rich spread

5. Stir fried scallops, broccoli and water chestnuts in black bean
sauce (purchase sauce at Asian market or health food store)
     Seaweed salad
     Steamed jasmine rice

BALANCING SNACKS

celery with hummus	rye or rice crackers with cucumber slices
grapes	goat cheese
pumpkin seeds	olives
baked blue-corn chips with mild bean dip	jicama marinated in lime and fresh cilantro
vegetable soup	fresh blueberries
pea soup	fresh grapefruit

Breakfast Suggestions to Reduce Signs of Dampness with Cold

1. Poached egg with steamed basmati rice, scallions, and cracked black pepper
   Green tea
2. Shrimp-vegetable omelet (two egg whites for every whole egg), parsley, minced onions, and shrimp)
   Green tea
3. Cooked hot quinoa with cinnamon, and walnuts
   Green tea
4. Sprouted rye or whole-rye bread
   Lox or other smoked fish, capers, thin slice onion
   Green tea
5. Hot cooked cream of rice cereal with pumpkin seeds
   Rice milk (optional)
   Green tea

TIP *To add a creamy flavor and texture to hot cereals, try melting in a small amount of rice cheese (found in health food stores). Other options include roasted pumpkin seeds, raw honey, or the naturally sweet herb stevia. Stevia helps to stabilize blood sugar. It is 100 to 400 times sweeter than sugar, depending on how it is extracted. I prefer the whole-leaf extract, which comes as a brown syrup. It is neutral and can be used by all patterns.*

Lunch Suggestions to Reduce Signs of Dampness with Cold

1. Vegetable-shrimp stir fry (mustard greens, daikon radish, and mushrooms stir fried in a small amount of canola oil with minced garlic, ginger, and red pepper flakes)
   Chicken-broth steamed basmati rice
   Miso broth with scallions
   (Vegetarian suggestion: Omit shrimp and add toasted sesame seeds to stir fry.)
2. Open-faced grilled chicken sandwich on rye bread
   Sautéed broccoli rabe in small amount garlic and olive oil
   (Vegetarian suggestion: Substitute curried lentil-vegetable stew for sandwich.)

3. Black bean soup seasoned with red pepper, cumin, onions, garlic, and black pepper
    Kale and turnips simmered in chicken broth, sautéed in olive oil and sprinkled with toasted mustard seeds

 TIP *If cooking beans from scratch, add kombu, wakame, or other sea vegetables to cooking water to moisten signs of dryness (build yin fluids) and reduce problems with gas.*

4. Sautéed salmon and greens (braise mustard greens and turnips in chicken broth and wine; sauté salmon in olive oil with minced garlic; combine together and add olive pieces; season with salt and cracked black pepper)
    (Vegetarian suggestion: Substitute red beans for beef.)
5. Grilled skinless chicken breast seasoned with minced garlic, rosemary, and cracked black pepper
    Broth-cooked brussels sprouts and pearl onions flavored with prepared mustard
    (Vegetarian suggestion: Substitute a legume veggie burger with grilled onions for chicken.)

Dinner Suggestions to Reduce Signs of Dampness with Cold

1. Cajun shrimp with red beans and rice (use Cajun spice mix to sauté jumbo shrimp in a small amount of canola oil; season beans with onion and chilies)
    Collard greens boiled in chicken broth
    (Vegetarian suggestion: Omit shrimp.)
2. Baked chicken seasoned with thyme, garlic, and capers
    Roasted parsnips, and carrots with parsley and olive oil
    Sautéed turnip greens
    (Vegetarian suggestion: Omit chicken and add pumpkin seeds to turnip greens.)
3. Vegetarian "burger" with grilled onions and mushrooms (choose legume-based, non soy burger), sliced dill pickle, prepared mustard
    Sautéed broccoli
    Sourdough rye bread
4. Grilled ahi tuna with ginger-sake marinade

Pan-sautéed pumpkin pieces (boil sweet cooking pumpkin or Japanese pumpkin [kobucha] until almost done; sear in olive oil and garlic)

Bok choy stir fried in canola oil with garlic and fish sauce (Vegetarian suggestion: Substitute egg flower soup for ahi tuna. Add black sesame seeds to pumpkin.)

5. Stir fried chicken and mixed vegetables (stir fry asparagus, parsnips, and onions in a small amount of canola oil, adding sake, broth, and tamari sauce to cook through)

Steamed basmati rice

BALANCING SNACKS

unsalted, dry-roasted almonds or walnuts	beef jerky
almond cheese and sliced onion on rye cracker	spicy pumpkin seeds
smoked salmon on rye toast	sourdough rye bread with spicy hummus
goat cheese	

DAMP-REDUCING COOKING METHODS

low-oil grilling	broiling
sautéing	convection-oven cooking
baking	boiling
roasting	simmering
barbecuing	pressure cooking

DRYING/DIURETIC HERBS AND SEASONINGS

basil	kelp
black pepper	kudzu (thickener)
dill weed	lemon/lime juice
dulse	parsley
caraway seeds	scallions

celery seeds

sea vegetables (dulse, wakame, hijiki—both diuretic and moistening)

coriander seeds

tamarind

honey, raw

vegetable broth

horseradish

white pepper

DRYING/DIURETIC TEAS AND BEVERAGES

black tea

green tea

buchu leaves

hibiscus

burdock root

nettles

calendula

oatstraw

coffee (warming initially but then cools and dehydrates the body)

parsley

catnip

raspberry leaf

cayenne

red clover blossoms

chamomile

rosehips

cleavers

sage

chrysanthemum flowers

spearmint

corn silk

uva ursi

dandelion leaf and root

(warming initially but then cools and dehydrates the body)

Several herbs can be combined to make a tasty fluid-balancing blend. For each cup of tea, pour boiling water over about a tablespoon of herb mix in a tea ball or teapot and let steep 3–5 minutes. Try a combination of uva ursi, fennel seed, red clover, corn silk, and spearmint.

19

MEAL SUGGESTIONS AND COOKING TIPS FOR REDUCING SIGNS OF DRYNESS AND FOR TONIFYING YIN

he following cooking suggestions and meal ideas can be helpful in balancing signs of dryness, including a dry parched throat and mouth, flushed cheeks, dry skin and hair, irritability, sugar cravings, and insomnia (see chapter seven). Healthy body fluids, including natural skin oils, moist mucous membranes, normal hormone production, and sufficient intestinal moisture for elimination, reflect the state of our yin fluids. Remember that moisture is relatively yin, and yin fluids come from balanced, healthy kidneys. Foods that moisten dryness are essentially those that enhance the health of our kidneys. They *tonify the yin,* according to TCM.

Because our moist, yin element diminishes with age, the following meal suggestions are beneficial at menopause or with advancing age. They are also helpful if you work or live in a dry climate or in a centrally-heated or air-conditioned building as well as if you are under stress and find yourself mentally ruminating, overly irritable, short tempered, or waking up hot in the night.

Cooling, moistening foods, especially lightly cooked vegetables, tofu, sea vegetables, black beans, millet, and cold-water fatty fish, are particularly helpful. Raw vegetables and fruits, although helpful for those with signs of heat, may be a problem for those with dryness because they can cause digestive problems.

Refined sugars, including candy, sweet breakfast cereals, baked sweets, ice cream, and frozen yogurt, aggravate the blood-sugar imbalances often experienced by those with a dry pattern. Adequate protein, especially from fish, soy, poultry, and eggs, reduces cravings for sugar while nourishing the kidneys, the source of yin fluids.

Guidelines to Moisten Dryness/Tonify the Yin

1. Relax more, especially in nature. Take walks near the ocean, a lake or stream, or in damp, wooded areas. Reduce stress.
2. Include two and a half to four cups of lightly cooked vegetables per day, including green beans, Napa cabbage, sea vegetables, sweet potatoes, and spinach. (Avoid raw vegetables and fruits if you have abdominal bloating or indigestion.)
3. Include an essential fat-rich food daily. Choose from fatty fish (such as salmon, mackerel, herring, and trout), pumpkin seeds, hemp seeds, almonds, sesame seeds, walnuts, or flaxseeds.
4. Include two servings of protein per day, preferably from the following: fish, shellfish, chicken, eggs, lean pork, black beans, soy products, or goat's milk cheese or yogurt.
5. Choose two or three servings of moistening whole grains per day, such as millet, sweet rice, or whole barley.
6. Reduce or avoid spicy foods, alcohol, coffee, sugar, hydrogenated vegetable oils, and other "bad" fats, as well as fat-free meals.
7. Increase sour and *full sweet foods*. Decrease bitter and pungent foods. Balance each of the five flavors.

TIP *The "sweet" flavor refers not only to empty sweets such as ice cream, cookies, and candy, but also to full sweets, including poultry, meats, seafood, fruit, root vegetables, and whole grains.*

Breakfast Suggestions for Moistening Dryness/Tonifying the Yin

1. Cooked millet cereal (cook with diced apple and nutmeg) with rice syrup, goat milk yogurt, and ground flax seeds
    Herb tea

 TIP *To flavor hot cereals, use moistening fruits or soy milk. For a delicious, creamy, savory hot cereal, try a mild melted soy cheese or goat's milk cheese. To sweeten your hot cereal or yogurt, use barley-malt syrup, maple syrup, or brown-rice syrup. To reduce refined sweets, try the naturally sweet herb stevia, which contains no calories and helps to stabilize blood sugar. It is 100 to 400 times sweeter than sugar, depending on how it is extracted. I prefer the whole-leaf extract, which comes as a brown syrup. It is neutral and can be used by all patterns. Just six to eight drops can sweeten a serving of cereal.*

2. Omelet (eggs, asparagus, tomato, goat cheese)
    Whole-wheat toast with omega-rich spread
    Soy milk
3. Soy sausage or soy cheese
    Poached egg(s)
    Whole-wheat sourdough toast with omega-rich spread
    Soy milk

4. Breakfast burrito (black beans, sweet rice, diced tomato, avocado, cumin, and soy cheese in whole-wheat tortilla)
    Soy milk

 TIP *If cooking beans from scratch, add kombu to cooking water to moisten signs of dryness (build yin fluids) and reduce problems with gas.*

5. Whole- or cracked-barley cereal, with sliced banana, plain yogurt and ground flaxseeds
    Herb tea

 TIP *Flax seeds are an excellent source of essential oils, fiber, and protein. When added to hot cereals, they provide a nutty, rich, grain-like texture and bulk. They are filling, provide moisture, stimulate elimination (alleviate constipation), and help stabilize blood-sugar levels.*

Lunch Suggestions for Moistening Dryness/Tonifying the Yin

1. Black-bean soup with melted cheese (soy or goat cheese is best)
   Green beans and oyster mushrooms sautéed in olive oil,
      adding broth and simmer until done
   Whole grain sourdough bread with omega-rich spread
   Herb tea or water

2. Stir fried tofu and vegetables (Napa cabbage, red bell peppers,
   carrots, and tofu stir fried in canola oil with oyster sauce, and
   sprinkled with toasted black sesame seeds)
   Steamed black rice with toasted sesame oil
   Miso soup
   Herb tea or water

3. Vegetable-barley soup (add fresh, sweet potatoes, green beans,
   parsnips and marjoram to canned soup, or make from scratch with
   chicken stock)
   Roast turkey, light and dark meat
   Sprouted- or whole-wheat bread with hummus, dill pick-
      le, and tomato slices
   (Vegetarian suggestion: Substitute melted soy or almond
      cheese for turkey.)
   Herb tea or water

4. Stir fried spinach with crab (crab, spinach, water chestnuts garlic,
   and ginger stir fried in canola oil and flavored with toasted sesame oil,
   ginger, garlic, fish sauce, miso paste, and toasted black sesame seeds)
   Steamed rice with sauce from stir fry
   (Vegetarian suggestion: Omit crab and add extra black
      sesame seeds.)
   Herb tea or water

5. Chicken-vegetable-barley soup
   Boiled beets and yams (boil beets and yams in chicken
      broth, drain, then add tarragon, juice of an orange,
      and butter)
   Seaweed salad
   (Vegetarian suggestion: Substitute navy bean soup for
      chicken-vegetable-barley.)
   Herb tea

Dinner Suggestions for Moistening Dryness/Tonifying the Yin

1. Salmon poached in rice wine, fish sauce, mushroom soy sauce, and fresh ginger slices

    Spinach sautéed in canola oil with garlic and soy sauce

    Sweet potato (boil until just done, slice, then grill in canola oil)

    (Vegetarian suggestion: Substitute tempeh for salmon.)

    Water or herb tea

2. Paella (sweet rice cooked in broth and clam juice with saffron and parsley; add your choice of chicken, mussels, clams, oysters, or cold water fatty fish)

    Asparagus sautéed in olive oil, flavored with balsamic vinegar

    (Vegetarian suggestion: Omit seafood and melt in a mild, fresh goat cheese or soy cheese.)

    Water or herb tea

3. Risotto (arborio rice cooked in broth, olive oil, asparagus, mushrooms, and tomatoes, with goat's milk romano cheese)

    Marinated sautéed tofu or tempeh (or use prepackaged flavored tofu)

    Ripe black or green olives

    Water or herb tea

4. Roast chicken marinated in white wine, rice vinegar, and miso paste

    Broth-cooked green beans with pine nuts and butter

    Hot whole barley with parsley, butter, sea salt, and white pepper

    (Vegetarian suggestion: Substitute tofu for chicken—use marinade listed above.)

    Water or herb tea

5. Pork loin braised in red wine, broth, and onions, and topped with capers

    Baked potato stuffed with butter or olive oil, melted soy cheese, and dulse flakes

    Beet greens sautéed in olive oil

    Pickled beets

    Water or herb tea

Many of these dishes or similar versions can be made from scratch, ordered at restaurants, or purchased ready-made. Be sure to check labels or ask about ingredients used in preparation. Depending on your body pattern, some of the ingredients you may want to avoid include dairy products, wheat, refined sugars, and meat products if you are a vegetarian. It is always best to avoid heavily sugared or salted foods, partially hydrogenated vegetable oils (including margarine), saturated fats (including lard) and polyunsaturated oils subjected to heat, either in processing or in cooking. That includes corn, safflower, sunflower, soybean, and cottonseed oils, as well as peanut oil, which may contain a mold toxin. I suggest using as few canned foods as possible. Canned products are boiled to the point of being sterile and sealed with no oxygen, leaving them devoid of vital energy, or Qi, which circulates readily through fresh foods.

BALANCING SNACKS

fresh figs and almonds

cantaloupe with goat yogurt
  sweetened with barley malt syrup

grapes and pumpkin seeds

pear or apple pieces and ripe aged, goat cheese

Greek, Spanish or Italian olives

soy cheese and sesame rice crackers

marinated anchovies or sardines with whole grain
  bread or crackers

MOISTENING COOKING METHODS

braising in broth, oil, or a combination

sautéing in oil

simmering

stewing or poaching in water, wine, or broth

MOISTENING/CALMING HERBS AND SEASONINGS

barley-malt syrup

basil

black sesame seeds, toasted

blackstrap molasses

marjoram

rice syrup

sea salt (in small amounts)

sea vegetables (dulse, wakame, hijiki—both diuretic
  and moistening)

dill weed   vegetable and poultry broth
honey, cooked

MOISTENING/CALMING HERBAL TEAS

catnip   nettles

chamomile   passionflower

hops   red clover

lemon balm   red raspberry

licorice   rose petals

marshmallow root   valerian

Several herbs can be combined into a tasty moistening blend. For each cup of tea, pour boiling water over about a tablespoon of herb mix in a tea ball or teapot and let steep 3–5 minutes. Try a combination of chamomile, rose petals, red clover, and licorice (use licorice sparingly if you have high blood pressure or are using steroid medications).

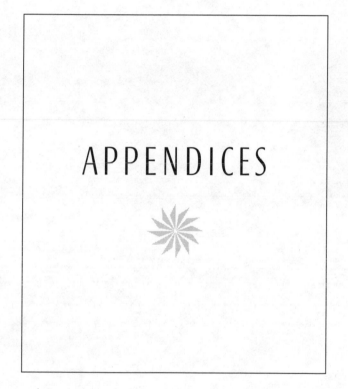

APPENDICES

APPENDIX A

GUIDELINES FOR
REDUCING SIGNS OF WIND

As described in chapter ten, wind signs include pains that move from place to place on the body, tremors, seizures, shaking, itchy patches on the skin, dizziness, stroke, and nervousness. These symptoms are generally accompanied by signs of heat, cold, or dampness; therefore, it is best to follow guidelines for balancing the pattern present with the wind signs. Avoid eggs, crab, coffee, and buckwheat, which tend to aggravate wind.

Beneficial foods for reducing signs of wind with cold include basil, fennel, ginger, anise seed, leeks, pine nuts, red-fleshed fish, and warming green leafy vegetables, plus the vegetables given below. Beneficial foods for reducing signs of wind with heat include all leafy greens—especially dandelion greens—Napa cabbage, soy products, and celery as well as the foods below.

Foods generally beneficial for wind include cabbage family vegetables (cabbage, kale, broccoli, cauliflower, brussels sprouts), chestnuts, asparagus, kale, mustard greens, beets, sage, whole or rolled oats, black sesame seeds, parsnips, turnips, coconut, flaxseeds, hemp seeds, fish, shrimp, beans, lentils, barley, millet, quinoa, and sweet rice.

APPENDIX B

GREEN TEA:
A BALANCING, HEALTH-PROMOTING
BEVERAGE FOR EVERYONE

Green tea is a soothing blend of bitter and sweet flavors. Sipped hot, it is refreshing and uplifting and can aid digestion, ease sugar cravings, and restore flagging energy levels. Studies show green tea may brighten and clear the skin, fight dental cavities, boost immunity, reduce risk of heart disease by lowering blood cholesterol and blood fats, and even prevent cancer. The disease-fighting, longevity-promoting potential of green tea is so significant that it has caught the attention of the National Cancer Institute and the National Institutes of Health, two mainstream sources of funding for the first US studies of green tea's effects on health.

In China and Japan, green tea is consumed throughout the day, including during and after meals. The fact that this beverage flows in Japan and China like Coca-Cola does in the United States is thought to contribute to the dramatically lower rates of heart disease and many cancers in Asia. These health-bestowing properties come from plant-based chemicals called polyphenols. Most of these phenols work as antioxidants, compounds that have been shown to slow diseases of aging, including heart disease, cataracts, and cancer, by slowing oxidation reactions (common but hazardous cellular reactions that can initiate cancer and the fatty buildup on artery walls). Antioxidants, also found in fruits and vegetables, prevent cholesterol from doing its damage by keeping it from sticking onto artery walls. Drinking green tea is associated with decreased harmful cholesterol and triglyceride levels and increased protective HDL cholesterol. One study looked at 1,371 Japanese men over age forty. Their LDL cholesterol and triglycerides dropped while their HDL rose when they drank green tea daily.[104]

One of the main polyphenols in green tea, called epigallocatechin gallate (EGCG), has been shown in laboratory studies to be a hundred times more effective than vitamin C and twenty-five times more powerful than vitamin E at protecting against harmful oxidation reactions. Other polyphenols in green tea have similar properties.[105] Japanese studies show EGCG specifically inhibits the growth of human lung cancer cells, perhaps one reason why Japanese men can smoke more than American men yet suffer less from lung cancer. Drinking green tea protects lung tissue, in particular, from hydroxyl radical and other oxidizing compounds generated by tobacco smoke. Researchers found green tea reduced lung tumor formation in mice by 50 percent.[106] The antioxidants in green tea appear to protect DNA from changes associated with cancer.

Apparently, the amount of tea one drinks is directly related to its effectiveness. People who drink more than three cups of green tea per day appear to stave off cancer longer than do those drinking fewer than three cups per day. In one controlled study of 8,552 individuals living in Japan, it was found that those consuming green tea had a lower incidence of cancer, particularly among females, and especially when participants drank more than ten cups of green tea per day.[107]

A regular intake of green tea may help keep you free of colds, the flu, and other infections. Tea appears to increase the activity of several infection-fighting white blood cells, including B and T lymphocytes, and natural killer cells.[108] Green tea also appears to protect the liver against toxins.[109] John Weisburger, PhD, of the American Health Foundation, recommends drinking four to five cups of green tea per day. Drinking more than four cups per day may substitute for up to two of the five to nine servings of vegetables and fruits recommended for health.

Tea has long been considered a fat-burner in Chinese medicine, both because it keeps the blood from getting thick and fatty from fat-rich foods and because it keeps fat burned off. When consumed along with large, fat-rich meals, it reduces the accumulation of fat in the blood and on sites of the body. In one study with rats, green tea was found to increase thermogenesis, the ability to burn fat and an indication of metabolic rate, 20 to 500 percent, depending on the dose.[110]

Black teas, such as Lipton, English Breakfast, and Earl Grey, are more common in Western cultures than are green or oolong teas. Black teas are warming and contain more caffeine than green. Black, oolong, and green teas come from the same plant, *Camellia sinenis*. The difference is that to make black tea, the leaves are dried, crushed, and fermented. Crushing releases enzymes that oxidize the leaves, leaving them black. Oolong teas, such as jasmine, are oxidized for a shorter period of time, leaving them lighter in color, sometimes even red. Green tea leaves, in contrast, are not crushed at all and therefore do not oxidize. Rather, the leaves are steamed, rolled, and then dried. Steaming prevents oxidation, leaving different chemical constituents from those found in fermented black tea leaves.

Green teas are as varied as coffees or wines. Loose leaves generally provide a higher quality tea than do the packaged tea bags available in grocery stores. Dragon's Well, cultivated in China's West Lake region, is considered one of the highest quality green teas. Gunpowder and silver tip are also flavorful Chinese green teas.

Green tea contains about forty milligrams of caffeine per cup, about half that of coffee. Black teas have slightly more. You can decaffeinate your tea by pouring off the water after steeping the leaves or bag a minute or so, then re-adding hot water—the caffeine is released in the first one to two minutes of steeping. However, the small amount of caffeine in green tea helps clear the mind and promotes alertness. Too much green tea, of course, and you may wind up overstimulated, as is the case with too much coffee. But because it has less caffeine than does coffee and it is in a form more slowly assimilated by the body, green tea provides a steadier release of energy and alertness than coffee's abrupt jolt.

According to TCM, green tea is slightly cooling, even when consumed hot. (Reddish-colored oolong or black Indian and English teas are more warming in nature.) The bitter property of green makes it beneficial to clearing mucous and phlegm from the body. Thus, it is a good choice for the morning, a time when we want to clear the foggy dampness that follows us from sleep. It is also ideal for stimulating digestion and clearing the heavy feeling created by mucous-forming meats and fatty foods. Green tea is beneficial for all patterns at any time (except when you are experiencing insomnia or anxiety); its cooling nature makes it particularly refreshing on hot summer days. Green tea is also said to "banish fatigue or fits of depression, raising the spirits and inducing a general feeling of well being."[111]

---

104. Weil, Andrew, "The Healing Power of Green Tea." *Dr Andrew Weil's Self-Healing Newsletter* (October 1998): 2.
105. Ibid., 2–3.
106. "Exploring the Chemopreventive Properties of Tea." *Primary Care and Cancer: American Health Foundation Update* 15(2) (February 1995): 30–31.
107. Imai, K. et al., "Cancer Preventive Effects of Drinking Green Tea Among a Japanese Population," *Preventive Medicine* 26 (1997): 769–775.
108. Weil, Andrew, "The Healing Power of Green Tea," *Dr Andrew Weil's Self-Healing Newsletter* (October 1998): 2–3.
109. Imai, K., and K. Nakachi, "Cross Sectional Study of Effects of Drinking Green Tea on Cardiovascular and Liver Diseases." *British Medical Journal* 310 (1995): 693–96.
110. Dullo, A.G., J. Seydoux, and L. Girardier, "Tealine and Thermogenesis: Interactions Between Polyphenols, Caffeine and Sympathetic Activity." *International Journal of Obesity* 20(S-4) (May 1996): 71.
111. Blonfeld, John, *The Chinese Art of Tea*. Shambhala (1985): 187.

APPENDIX C

A FEW COOKING IDEAS, SUGGESTED FLAVORINGS, AND RECOMENDED FOOD BRANDS

Congee

When I was in China, breakfast always included a bowl of *congee* or *jook*. This hot, soupy porridge consisted of a grain, usually rice, cooked with some sort of poultry, meat, or bean, or sometimes red dates or vegetables. It is made by cooking one part grain with five to six parts water and a pinch of salt. Cooking time is the key. The mixture is cooked for four hours to as long as overnight. The longer it cooks, the more powerful the effects on strengthening the spleen and thus digestion.

I recommend congee to my clients who are weakened from an illness or from surgery as well as those with digestive problems, including irritable bowel syndrome, colitis, or Crohn's disease. Congee is tonifying in Chinese medicine and thus good for rebuilding the body tissues. It helps restore yin fluids and can benefit a pattern of dryness. When made with beans or vegetables, congee cools a pattern of heat. When made with meat or spices, congee becomes warming.

Broken Bone "Longevity" Soup

Broken bone soup is rich in minerals and other nutrients from bone and its marrow center. Our Western understanding of the properties of a bone-infused broth (or soup) is that it is rich in calcium, magnesium, and the other minerals in bone. TCM describes a healing essence from the bone marrow exposed to the simmering broth. This marrow essence is thought to be particularly beneficial for growth in young children as well as in restoring depleted kidney yin from stress, age, or poor diet. Use the following recipe.

2 lbs. organic beef, veal, and/or chicken bones (may be bones reserved from cooking soup or stew)
1 onion
1 carrot
2 stalks celery
1 Tbs. apple cider vinegar
water to cover bones

If using raw bones with meat, place them in large stockpot with enough cold water to cover. Bring to boil and simmer until meat is tender (one to two hours).

Remove bones and meat. Chill cooking liquid at least five hours and remove congealed fat on surface.

When bones are cool, remove meat from them and use for another dish. Wrap cooked, cooled, meat-free bones (the ones you have just cooked or those from another roasted or stewed meat or poultry dish) in butcher paper or plastic bag and then newspaper. Place on hard, firm surface (a large stone, your driveway, or a cement walkway) and hit with hammer until bones are crushed enough to expose much of the marrow. Bones need not be reduced to fragments.

Return crushed bones to de-fatted cooking broth. Add water if necessary to cover bones by several inches. Add vegetables and simmer twelve to fifteen hours, adding water if necessary.

Strain through cheesecloth or fine strainer. Season with sea salt, and drink daily as a broth or make into a soup.

Greens

One of the most important healing foods is the broad category of leafy green vegetables. As green is considered the master color, greens benefit all body patterns. Most greens tend to be cooling and cleansing to body tissues, excellent for weight loss, calming the liver, reducing tension and anger. Those with signs of cold or who are underweight can bring warmth to a dish of greens by cooking them with garlic and ginger and serving them with warming meat or poultry dishes. The following suggestions are balanced for most body patterns and can be served with appropriate foods to add warmth or cooling properties as needed.

Quick Cooking Greens: spinach, Swiss chard, beet greens, bok choy, asparagus, pea sprouts, watercress, Napa cabbage, Chinese broccoli

Quick-cooking greens can be sautéed or stir-fried in two to five minutes, depending on how you like them. To retain bright green color, blanch greens first in boiling water one to two minutes. Drain and stir fry or sauté in small amount of oil until done. Or heat wok or skillet until hot, add a small amount of oil to coat pan, then add washed and torn or chopped raw leaves and cook, stirring, until tender.

Longer-Cooking Greens: Collard greens, mustard greens, turnip greens, kale, Russian kale, dandelion greens, brussels sprouts

To retain their bright color and to speed the cooking process, blanch these heartier greens in boiling water five to ten minutes, depending on how coarse they are, then plunge into cold water. Collard greens may require longer cooking, from twenty to forty-five minutes in boiling water, depending on how mature they are. Some recipes call for collard greens to be cooked as long as two hours. The shorter the cooking time, the more nutrients are retained. Drain, then sauté, braise or stir fry them.

IDEAS FOR COOKING GREENS FOR ALL BODY PATTERNS

Stir fry Chinese broccoli and water chestnuts in a hot wok with canola oil. Add oyster sauce to taste.

Heat wet, mixed young tender braising greens in covered pot until wilted. Drain and squeeze dry. Sauté minced garlic, then add greens and toasted pine nuts and sauté briefly.

Simmer bite-sized pieces of broccoli and sweet potatoes in a small amount of chicken broth until tender. Drain and drizzle with sesame oil, soy sauce, and toasted sesame seeds.

De-stem and chop collard greens. Sauté chopped onion until soft. Add collards and enough broth to cover. Simmer with mustard seeds until tender (20–45 minutes).

Brush asparagus and radicchio with olive oil, then grill (under broiler or on barbecue).

Sauté red onion in olive oil. Add washed torn spinach leaves and heat until wilted. Add lemon juice and crumbled feta cheese.

Sauté Swiss chard in olive oil until tender. Add splash of balsamic vinegar and sprinkle with rinsed capers.

Stir fry baby bok choy with sliced shiitake mushrooms until just soft. Stir in black bean sauce.

Cook chopped raw kale leaves into vegetable or chicken soup.

Simmer kale and mustard greens until tender. Add can of favorite soup.

Sauté washed, torn spinach leaves, and sliced mushrooms in olive oil. Add scrambled eggs.

Add chopped Napa cabbage leaves to simmering red beans during last five minutes of cooking.

Add broccoli or asparagus pieces to last three minutes of cooking rice or pasta.

Ideas for Sauces and Flavorings

Keep your kitchen stocked with a variety of sauces and flavorings; experiment with them and you will never grow tired of a vegetable-rich, healthful diet. Used in small amounts, the following flavorings are acceptable for any body pattern.

Balsamic Vinegar: A softly sweet, sour Italian specialty vinegar particularly good on cooked or raw greens or grilled vegetables and in marinades for chicken or beef. Delicious when used with a high-quality olive oil on grilled vegetables or sautéed greens. A high-quality balsamic vinegar is good to have around when you want to add a rich, powerful flavor to a dish. *(warming, moistening)*

Black Bean Sauce: This salty, fermented black bean paste can be used in a variety of cooked Chinese dishes. Use a small amount to flavor chicken, fish, shrimp, or vegetable Chinese stir fry dishes. Dilute with a small amount of broth. *(neutral, moistening)*

Broth (Chicken, Beef, or Vegetable): An excellent flavor enhancer when used instead of water for cooking savory dishes. Low sodium broths are available for those who should reduce salt. Broth imparts flavor plus nutrients to cooked vegetables, poultry, and fish. Poach fish in broth with lemon and wine. Simmer or steam vegetables in broth. Pour broth over a baked potato. Sauté chicken or beef, then add broth to finish cooking. Cook broccoli, cauliflower, or brussels sprouts in a small amount of broth rather than over a steamer; then use or drink the broth. (*beef—warming; chicken—neutral; vegetable—cooling, moisture-regulating*)

Coconut Milk: Found in canned or frozen versions, low-fat or regular, coconut milk is a purée of fresh coconut meat. It makes a delicious base for curried dishes or with lemon grass, kaffir leaves, and other Thai flavorings. (*neutral, moistening*)

Fish Sauce or Nuoc Mam: A basic Vietnamese flavoring made from the brine of pickled fish. This thin liquid adds saltiness and depth to sauces, fulfilling much the same function as soy sauce in cooking, yet with a unique flavor all its own. Use small amounts as a basic seasoning with coconut or citrus dishes, or as a replacement for soy sauce or in cooked dishes ranging from vegetables to fish or chicken. Diluted, it can be used as a dipping sauce. (*neutral*)

Kudzu: A Japanese powdered white starchy root used for thickening sauces or soups. Dissolve it in cold water, then pour into simmering sauce or soup. Kudzu tea is beneficial for relieving an upset stomach, renewing strength and vitality, and alleviating colds and flu. It is also used as a treatment for an excessive appetite and alcohol cravings. (*cooling to the stomach*)

Mirin: A sweet, syrupy Japanese cooking sherry made from rice. A flavorful addition along with soy sauce to braised, boiled, or stir fry dishes of vegetables, chicken, fish, or shellfish. Okay for all body patterns in small amounts. (*warming, moistening*)

Miso: This thick paste of fermented soy beans is useful for adding depth and richness to sauces without adding fat. It makes a delicious clear soup, ideal for a snack or sipped before a meal to reduce appetite. When used in sauces, it should be added to liquid after cooking to impart extra flavor to vegetables, meats, poultry, and fish. It is available in pale yellow, white, red ,or darker brown versions, depending on whether it was made with rice, barley, or other ingredients. As with other fermented products, miso is beneficial to digestion and the growth of "good" gut bacteria. *(neutral)*

Mustard (Prepared): Use any of the many varieties of mustards (champagne, dill, pepper, honey, and spicy) to add flavor to poultry, fish, or vegetables. Brussels sprouts are excellent simmered in vegetable or chicken broth flavored with a small amount of mustard and thickened with kudzu. Smear salmon filets with a layer of mustard, then grill or broil them. *(hot, drying)*

Mustard Seeds: These tiny yellow seeds add a delicious pungent flavor and crackly texture to any cooked dish, but in particular when used on cooked greens, cauliflower, or green beans. Toast them a few seconds in a hot skillet before sprinkling them on foods. *(hot, drying)*

Oyster Sauce: A slightly sweet and pungent sauce made with extract of oysters, salt, sugar, and a thickener. Delicious over Chinese broccoli or other greens. Excellent in stir fry dishes or sautéed vegetables. *(warming, moistening)*

Ponzu: Made from bitter orange rind, this sour yet tangy vinegary sauce makes a delicious dip for grilled poultry or seafood. *(neutral, moistening)*

Shaoxing Wine: A famous aged Chinese rice wine with a rich full flavor and aroma. This amber-colored liquid is often used in sauces or marinades for fish. *(warming)*

Rice Vinegar: A mild, tangy vinegar ideal for adding a sour note to vegetable dishes and salads. All three varieties can be used to flavor cooked dishes and serve as excellent additions for marinades; the white variety, however, is most often used for sweet dishes, the red as a dipping sauce, and the black for braising and in stir-fry dishes. *(warming, moistening)*

Sake: This Japanese rice wine adds flavor to boiled, stir fried, and one-pot dishes. Use in small amounts to finish a dish. *(warming)*

Soy Sauce: This versatile, dark, rich sauce adds flavor to almost any food. It can be used plain as a dip or in stir fry dishes and marinades for chicken, meat, fish, or vegetable dishes. It is made by fermenting soybeans, generally with wheat, plus salt and water. Soy sauce comes in mild to rich-tasting and light to dark varieties and can be flavored with mushrooms, shrimp, oysters, or other flavorings. *(neutral, moistening)*

Tamari or Shoyu Sauce: Basically the same as soy sauce, tamari, or shoyu sauce, is a thicker, richer version. It was traditionally made without wheat although now there are varieties on the market with wheat. Choose the wheat-free version if there are signs of dampness. *(neutral, moistening)*

Toasted Sesame Oil: An extremely flavorful, nutty-tasting oil, perfect in minute amounts to flavor vegetable, poultry, or meat dishes once they are cooked. A few drops on freshly steamed broccoli and sweet potatoes, along with some soy sauce, makes an excellent vegetable dish. Because only small amounts are needed, it a useful oil for all patterns. *(warming, moistening)*

Toasted Sesame Seeds: When toasted in a hot, dry pan on the stove until they begin to pop, sesame seeds add a spectacular, nutty flavor and crackly texture to vegetable dishes, salads, rice, and meat, poultry, and fish dishes. Try toasted black sesame seeds over stir fried broccoli with soy sauce and toasted sesame oil. Black sesame seeds are excellent for dryness. *(neutral, moistening)*

RECOMENDED SOY-BASED DAIRY ALTERNATIVES

WholeSoy Creamy Cultured Soy (Yogurt substitute)

White Wave Silk Plain Soymilk

Wildwood Plain Soymilk

Soyfresh Unswetened Soy Beverage

Wildwood Meltables (cheese substitute)

Tofu Rella by Rella Good Cheese Co. (cheese substitute)

Soya Kaas (cheese substitute)

RECOMMENDED RICE BASED "DAIRY" SUBSTITUTES

Vegan Rella by Rella Good Cheese Co.
Soyco Rice Cheese
Soyco Rice Butter

RECOMMENDED BUTTER/MARGARINE SUBSTITUTES

Spectrum Naturals Spread or Essential Omega Spread
Canoleo Margarine
Soyco Rice Butter

RECOMMENDED OILS

Spectrum Naturals
Hain
other cold or expeller-pressed organic oils

MAYONNAISE

Spectrum Naturals Lite Canola Mayo

STEVIA-BASED SWEETENERS

NuNaturals Stevia Powder or Extract (liquid or powder)
Planetary Formulas Stevia Whole Leaf Extract
NOW Stevia Extract

APPENDIX D

FINDING AN OMD OR AN ACUPUNCTURIST

Licensed acupuncturists (LAcs), Oriental Medical Doctors (OMDs), and Doctors of Oriental Medicine (DOMs) are among the professionals trained in traditional Chinese medical techniques, including acupuncture and medicinal herbs, to diagnose and treat patients. They may or may not recommend dietary changes, depending on their education and treatment philosophy. Most states require certification and licensure of these professionals; however, each state determines its own requirements for a degree and the title granted. Before selecting a practitioner, consumers should check their state's education and licensing requirements through their state's acupuncture board or acupuncture association.

Practitioners using OMD after their name may have received this advanced training in California in the 80s, a program that has since been phased out. Some practitioners trained in China use OMD to indicate doctorate status granted in that country. A nationally approved doctorate program is in the development stages in the US and is expected to be available to acupuncture students in the next few years. In order to find a qualified practitioner, contact your state acupuncture board or association or consult the American Association of Oriental Medicine (AAOM), the umbrella organization representing the acupuncture profession in the United States.

The American Association of Oriental Medicine (AAOM)
433 Front Street, Catasauqua, PA 18032
Tel: 888.500.7999
Web site: www.aaom.org

ACKNOWLEDGMENTS

Writing this book opened my eyes to the necessity of others to our successes, especially accomplishments built on knowledge. The perfect teachers, practitioners, clients, researchers, healers, and friends materialized just as they were needed with just the right gem of insight, research finding, healing tool, or source of support.

Thank you, Glenn, for waiting for me through hours of manuscript writing, for acknowledging and respecting the importance of this work, and for taking your herbs. I thank my parents for trusting my career and education decisions and supporting me as I wound through the maze of understanding nutrition and healing.

I deeply appreciate the long yin-depleting hours Sarah Baldwin put in as my editor. In her determination to understand every facet of this material she applied the principles of the book to balance her own pattern. I thank Ellen Cavalli for her editorial work and in smoothly passing off the manuscript to

Sarah. I thank Peter Beren, my agent, for securing a contract with my publisher and for his expertly crafted synopsis of the book in doing so.

I am grateful for the opportunity to work with Matthew Lore, my editor at Marlowe & Company, who not only understands and uses the healing power of nutrition and Chinese medicine in his own life, but is a master at marketing it to others.

I am extremely blessed by having teachers with profound wisdom, open minds, and a passion for understanding their areas of expertise. This includes Alan Gaby, MD, Jonathan Wright, MD, and Richard Kunin, MD, three brilliant medical doctors all confident and intelligent enough to effectively use foods and nutrients (instead of drugs and surgery) as therapies to heal illness, despite government and peer pressure to follow the conventional model. Thank you for all you do.

I am honored and thankful to be able to work with a great master of Chinese medicine from China, Dr. Yu Min Chen, OMD, LAc Thank you, Dr. Chen, for teaching me to understand body patterns and the balancing power of food from an Eastern perspective. I am also grateful for the acupuncture you've provided to help me stay in balance when emotionally and physically challenged.

I also wish to thank Dr. Yen Wei Choong, LAc, for introducing me to Chinese philosophy and medicine and helping me to understand the body and health from a new perspective.

Paul Pitchford has been an invaluable source of wisdom and knowledge of the Eastern principles of food and healing and a living example of balance. I am deeply grateful for his brilliant book, *Healing with Whole Foods*, and his patience and devotion as a teacher and healer.

I wish to express my gratitude to all my clients, to all you who have trusted me, challenged me, and showed me the awesome power of nutrition in healing and creating balance. And finally, I am eternally thankful for the higher power that works mysteriously through each of us, enabling us to heal and teach others, to experience life through our emotions, and to accomplish all we do in our lives.

ABOUT THE AUTHOR

With specialties in nutrition for energy, healing, balance, craving control and weight loss, Linda Prout, M.S., has nearly twenty years of experience in nutrition consulting, speaking and writing. The resident nutritionist at the Claremont Resort and Spa in Berkeley, California, she received her Bachelor of Science in Dietetics from the University of California at Davis and Master of Science in Nutrition from the University of Bridgeport, Connecticut. She has training in Asian medicine from Meiji College in San Francisco as well as from studying with oriental medicine doctors in China and the U.S. She has studied nutrient therapy with Western oriented ortho-molecular physicians. She is a consultant and speaker to corporations seeking to enhance employee productivity through lifestyle changes, as well as a counselor to individuals—including CEOs, attorneys, sales professionals, physicians, psychotherapists, teenagers, and new moms—seeking more energy and better health. She also serves as a consultant to the Discovery Health Channel. She lives in Santa Rosa, California.

INDEX